CLINICAL SKILLS FOR MEDICAL STUDENTS

Life is short, the art long, opportunity fleeting,

experiment treacherous, judgement difficult.

Hippocrates (c. 460–370 BC). Aphorisms, Aph. 1.

CLINICAL SKILLS FOR MEDICAL STUDENTS

Sheheryar Kabraji

Clinical Fellow in Medicine, Harvard Medical School, Boston
Resident in Medicine, Massachusetts General Hospital, Boston

AND

Neel Burton

Medical Student Tutor, Green Templeton College,
University of Oxford

Scion

This book, for US medical students, is an adaptation of *Clinical Skills for OSCEs, 4th edition* (ISBN 978 1 904842 82 8) first published in 2011.

First edition © Neel Burton, 2012
First edition published in 2012 by Scion Publishing Ltd

ISBN 978 1 904842 72 9

A CIP catalogue record for this book is available from the British Library.

Scion Publishing Limited
The Old Hayloft, Vantage Business Park, Bloxham Road, Banbury, Oxfordshire OX16 9UX, UK
www.scionpublishing.com

Important Note from the Publisher

The information contained within this book was obtained by Scion Publishing Limited from sources believed by us to be reliable. However, while every effort has been made to ensure its accuracy, no responsibility for loss or injury whatsoever occasioned to any person acting or refraining from action as a result of information contained herein can be accepted by the authors or publishers.

Although every effort has been made to ensure that all owners of copyright material have been acknowledged in this publication, we would be pleased to acknowledge in subsequent reprints or editions any omissions brought to our attention.

Readers should remember that medicine is a constantly evolving science and while the authors and publishers have ensured that all dosages, applications and practices are based on current indications, there may be specific practices which differ between communities. You should always follow the guidelines laid down by the manufacturers of specific products and the relevant authorities in the country in which you are practicing.

The pronoun 'he' has been used throughout the book, but this is for simplicity rather than implying a gender bias.

Typeset by Phoenix Photosetting, Chatham, Kent, UK
Printed by Henry Ling, Dorchester, UK

Contents

VIII. OBSTETRICS, GYNECOLOGY, AND SEXUAL HEALTH

IX. ORTHOPEDICS AND RHEUMATOLOGY

X. PAIN CONTROL

XI. COMMUNICATION SKILLS

Clinical Skills for Medical Students is the US edition and adaptation of *Clinical Skills for OSCEs*, an immensely popular textbook on clinical skills that is used in the UK and the world over. The book's core aim is to equip medical students and junior trainees with the skills to succeed in clinical practice. Its unique advantage is to provide detailed but concise step-by-step instructions not only on history-taking and physical examination, but also on other clinical skills – such as venepuncture or nasogastric intubation – that are seldom found in other textbooks.

Clinical Skills for Medical Students includes special boxes headed 'Junior Resident's Tips' and 'Senior Resident's Questions' that are designed to focus your attention on important and/or frequently tested areas. Also included for the first time are the published likelihood ratios for key clinical findings, which reflect the diagnostic power (or lack thereof) of an individual clinical finding.

We hope that our little book may serve as your guide and companion as you prepare for a lifetime in clinical practice. Please do get in touch to tell us how it might be improved in its next edition.

Ars longa, vita brevis. The art is long; life all too short.

Sheheryar Kabraji
Neel Burton
April 2012

neelburton@yahoo.com

Acknowledgment

Thanks go to Zach Wallace for his help with reading the proofs.

- **Don't panic.** Be philosophical about your exams. Put them into perspective. And remember that as long as you do your bit, you are statistically very unlikely to fail. Book a vacation to a sunny Caribbean island starting on the day after your exams to help focus your attention.

- **Read the instructions carefully and stick to them.** Sometimes it's just possible to have revised so much that you no longer 'see' the instructions and just fire out the bullet points like an automatic gun. If you forget the instructions or the actor looks at you like Caliban in the mirror, ask to read the instructions again. A related point is this: pay careful attention to the facial expression of the actor or examiner. Just as an ECG monitor provides live indirect feedback on the heart's performance, so the actor or examiner's facial expression provides live indirect feedback on your performance, the only difference being – I'm sure you'll agree – that facial expressions are far easier to read than ECG monitors.

- **Quickly survey the room for the equipment and materials provided.** You can be sure that items such as hand disinfectant, a reflex hammer, a sharps bin, or a box of Kleenex are not just random objects that the examiner later plans to take home.

- **First impressions count.** You never get a second chance to make a good first impression. As much of your future career depends on it, make sure that you get off to an early start. And who knows? You might even fool yourself.

- **Prefer breadth to depth.** Scores are normally distributed across a number of relevant domains, such that you will score higher for touching upon a large number of domains than for exploring any one domain in great depth. Do this only if you have time, if it seems particularly relevant, or if you are specifically asked. Perhaps ironically, touching upon a large number of domains makes you look more focused, and thereby safer and more competent.

- **Don't let examiners put you off or hold you back.** If examiners are present and are being difficult, that's their problem, not yours. Or at least, it's everyone's problem, not yours. And remember that all that is gold does not glitter; a difficult examiner may be a hidden gem.

- **Be genuine.** This is easier said than done, but then even actors are people. By convincing yourself that the OSCE stations are real situations, you are much more likely to score highly with the actors, if only by 'remembering' to treat them like real patients. This may hand you a merit over a pass and, in borderline situations, a pass over a fail. Although they never seem to think so, students usually fail OSCEs through poor communications skills and lack of empathy, not through lack of studying and poor memory.

- **Enjoy yourself.** After all, you did choose to be there, and you probably chose wisely. If you do badly in one station, try to put it behind you. It's not for nothing that psychiatrists refer to 'repression' as a 'defense mechanism', and a selectively bad memory will do you no end of good.

- **Keep to time but do not appear rushed.** If you don't finish by the first bell, complete those crucial parts of the history and exam that are most relevant to the chief complaint. Then summarize and conclude.

- **Be nice to the patient.** Have I already said this? Introduce yourself, shake hands, smile, even joke if it seems appropriate – it makes life easier for everyone, including yourself. Remember to explain everything to the patient as you go along, to ask him about pain before you touch him, and to thank him on the second bell. The patient holds the key to the station, and he may hand it to you on a silver platter if you seem deserving enough. That having been said, if you reach the end of the station and feel that something is amiss, there's no harm in gently reminding him, for example, "Is there anything else that you feel is important but that we haven't had time to talk about?" Nudge-nudge.

- **Take a step back to jump further.** Last minute cramming is not going to magically turn you into a good doctor, so spend the day before the exam relaxing and sharpening your mind. Go to the beach, play some sports, rent a DVD. And make sure that you are tired enough to fall asleep by a reasonable hour.

- **Finally, remember to practice, practice, and practice.** Look at the bright side of things: at least you're not going to be alone, and there are going to be plenty of opportunities for good conversations, good laughs, and good meals. You might even make lifelong friends in the process. And then go off to that Caribbean island.

Hand washing

Hands must be washed before every episode of care that involves direct contact with a patient's skin, their food or medication, invasive devices, or dressings, and after any activity or contact that potentially contaminates the hands.

The procedure

- Remove your watch and any jewelry that you may be wearing, or indicate that you would do so.
- Roll up your sleeves.
- Turn on the hot and cold taps with your elbows and wait until the water is warm.
- Thoroughly wet your hands.
- Apply liquid soap or disinfectant from the dispenser. Liquid soap is used in most hospital situations. Disinfectants include aqueous chlorhexidine ('Hibiscrub') and povidone iodine ('Betadine'). Alcohol hand rubs offer a practical alternative to liquid soaps and disinfectants, but simple soap bars should be avoided.
- Wash your hands using the Ayliffe hand washing technique (see *Figure 1* overleaf):
  ① palm to palm
  ② right palm over left dorsum and left palm over right dorsum
  ③ palm to palm with fingers interlaced
  ④ back of fingers to opposing palms with fingers interlocked
  ⑤ rotational rubbing of right thumb clasped in left palm and left thumb clasped in right palm
  ⑥ rotational rubbing, backward and forward, with clasped fingers of right hand in left palm and clasped fingers of left hand in right palm.
- Rinse your hands thoroughly.
- Turn the taps off with your elbows.
- Dry your hands with a paper towel and discard it in the foot-operated bin, remembering to use the pedal rather than your clean hands. If using alcohol gel allow to air dry before patient contact. Remember that washing with soap and water is required after coming into contact with patients with certain precautions e.g. *C. difficile*.
- Consider applying an emollient.

General skills and procedures

Station 1 Hand washing

1.1

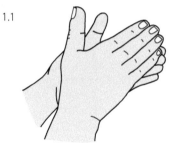

1.2

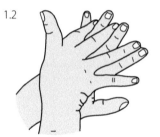

1.3

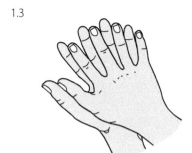

1.4

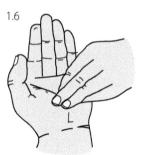

1.5

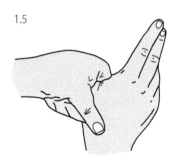

1.6

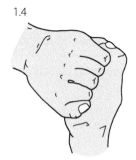

Figure 1. Ayliffe hand washing technique:
   1.1 Palm to palm
   1.2 Right palm over left dorsum and left palm over right dorsum
   1.3 Palm to palm fingers interlaced
   1.4 Backs of fingers to opposing palms with fingers interlocked
   1.5 Rotational rubbing of right thumb clasped in left palm and vice versa
   1.6 Rotational rubbing, backward and forward with clasped fingers of right hand in left palm and vice versa

Scrubbing up for the operating room

> **The equipment:** Operating rooms may vary in available equipment and routine. As always, scrub nurses know best but the scheme below should provide a framework that can be adapted to local protocol.

- Scrubs.
- Clogs or plastic overshoes.
- Surgical cap.
- Face mask.

- Sterile gown pack.
- Sterile gloves.
- Brush packet containing a nail brush and nail pick.

Before handwashing

State that you would:

- Change into scrubs.
- Put on clogs or plastic overshoes.
- Don a surgical cap, tucking all your hair underneath it.
- Remove all items of jewelry, including your watch.
- Enter the scrubbing room.
- Put on a face mask, and ensure that it covers both your nose and mouth.
- Open a sterile gown pack *without touching the gown*.
- Lay out a pair of sterile gloves *without touching the gloves*.

Handwashing

- Open a brush packet containing a nail brush and nail pick.
- Turn on the hot and cold taps and wait until the water is warm.

 From here on, keep your hands above your elbows at all times.

The social wash

- Wash your hands with liquid disinfectant, either chlorhexidine ('Hibiscrub') or povidone iodine ('Betadine'), lathering up your arms to 2 cm above the elbows.

The second wash

- Use the nail pick from the brush packet to clean under your fingernails.
- Dispense soap on to the sponge side of the brush and use the sponge to scrub from your fingertips to 2 cm above your elbows (30 seconds per arm).

 Dispense soap using your elbow or a foot pedal, not your hands.

- To rinse, start from your hands and move down to your elbows so that the rinse water does not re-contaminate your hands.

The third wash

- Using the brush side of the brush, scrub your fingernails (30 seconds per arm).

- Using the sponge side of the brush, scrub:
  - each finger and interdigital space in turn (30 seconds per arm)
  - the palm and back of your hands (30 seconds per arm)
  - your forearms, moving up circumferentially to 2 cm above your elbows (30 seconds per arm)

 Remember to keep the brush well-soaped at all times.

- To rinse, start from your hands and move down to your elbows.
- Turn the taps off with your elbows.

After handwashing

- Use the towels in the gown pack to dry your arms from the fingertips down.
- Pick up the gown from the inside and shake it open, ensuring that it does not touch anything.
- Put your arms through the sleeves, but do not put your hands through the cuffs.
- Put on the gloves without touching the outside of the gloves. Practice this – it's not easy!
- Ask an assistant to tie up the gown for you.

 After scrubbing up, keep your hands in front of your chest and do not touch any non-sterile areas, including your mask and hat.

Venepuncture/phlebotomy

Specifications: An OSCE station may consist of an anatomical arm and all the equipment that might be required. Assume that the anatomical arm is a patient and take blood from it.

Before starting

- Introduce yourself to the patient.
- Explain the procedure and ask for his consent to carry it out. For example, *"I would like to take a blood sample from you to check how your kidneys are working. This is a quick, simple, and routine procedure which involves inserting a small needle into one of the veins on your arm. You will feel a sharp scratch when the needle is inserted, and there may be a little bit of bleeding afterwards. Do you have any questions?".*
- Ask him which arm he prefers to have blood taken from.
- Ask him to expose this arm.
- Gather the equipment in a tray.

The equipment
In a tray, gather: - A pair of non-sterile gloves. - A tourniquet. - Alcohol wipes. - A 21G (green) needle and Vacutainer holder. - The bottles appropriate for the tests that you are sending for (these vary from hospital to hospital, but are generally yellow for biochemistry, purple for hematology, pink for group and save and crossmatch, blue for clotting, grey for glucose, and black for ESR). - Cotton swabs.

 Make sure you have a sharps box close at hand.

The procedure

- Wash your hands (see *Station 1*).
- Position the patient so that his arm is fully extended. Ensure that he is comfortable.
- Apply the tourniquet.
- Select a vein by palpation: the bigger and straighter the better. The vein selected is most commonly the median cubital vein in the antecubital fossa.
- Don a pair of non-sterile gloves.
- Clean the venepuncture site using the alcohol swabs. Explain that the alcohol swabs may feel a little cold.
- Once the alcohol has dried off, attach the needle to the Vacutainer holder.
- Tell the patient to expect a 'sharp scratch'.
- Retract the skin to stabilize the vein and insert the needle into the vein.
- Keeping the needle still, place a Vacutainer tube on the needle-holder and let it fill.
- Once all the necessary tubes are filled, release the tourniquet. Remember that the tubes need to be filled in a certain order.
- Release the tourniquet.

- Remove the needle from the vein and apply pressure on the puncture site.
- Dispose of the needle in the sharps box.
- Remove and dispose of the gloves in the clinical waste bin.

After the procedure

- Ensure that the patient is comfortable.
- Thank the patient.
- Label the tubes (at least: patient's name, date of birth, and hospital number; date and time of blood collection).
- Fill in the blood request form (at least: patient's name, date of birth, and hospital number; date of blood collection; tests required).
- Document the blood tests that have been ordered in the patient's notes.

Junior Resident's tips

If the veins are not apparent

- Lower the arm over the bedside.
- Ask the patient to exercise his arm by repeatedly clenching his fist.
- Gently tap the venepuncture site with two fingers.
- Apply a warm compress to the venepuncture site.
- Do not cause undue pain to the patient by trying over and over again – call a more experienced co-worker instead.
- Use femoral or radial stab as a last resort.

In the event of a needlestick injury

- Encourage bleeding, wash with soap and running water.
- Immediately report the injury to your hospital's infection control office and go to the emergency department for further evaluation.
- If there is a significant risk of HIV, post-exposure prophylaxis should be started as soon as possible.
- Fill out an incident form.

For more information on the management of needlestick injury, refer to local or national protocols.

Peripheral intravenous access and setting up an infusion

As a house officer you will often have to place an intravenous catheter and sometimes start a drip without an infusion pump. This chapter covers both scenarios.

Before starting

- Introduce yourself to the patient.
- Explain the procedure and ask for his consent to carry it out. For example, *"I would like to insert a thin plastic tube into one of the veins on your arm. The tube will enable you to receive intravenous fluids and prevent you from becoming dehydrated. You may feel a sharp scratch when the tube is inserted. Do you have any questions?"*
- Ask him which arm he would prefer to have the catheter on.
- Ask him to expose this arm.
- Gather the equipment in a tray.

 It is important to read the instructions for the station carefully. If, for example, the instructions specify that the patient is under general anesthesia, you are probably not going to gain any marks for explaining the procedure.

Intravenous access only

The equipment
In a tray, gather: • A pair of non-sterile gloves. • A tourniquet. • Alcohol swabs. • An intravenous catheter of appropriate size (*Table 1*). Size is primarily determined by the viscosity of the fluid to be infused and the required rate of infusion. • A pre-filled 5 ml syringe containing saline flush. • Adhesive tape. • A sharps box.

The procedure

- Wash your hands (see *Station 1*).
- Position the patient so that his arm is fully extended. Ensure that he is comfortable.
- Apply the tourniquet.
- Select a vein by palpation: the bigger and straighter the better. The dorsum of the hand and the antecubital fossa are common sites but can be awkward for patient comfort.
- Don a pair of non-sterile gloves.
- Clean the skin with an alcohol swab and let it dry.
- Remove the intravenous catheter from its packaging and remove its cap.
- Tell the patient to expect a 'sharp scratch'.
- Anchor the vein by stretching the skin and insert the catheter and needle at an angle of approximately 30 degrees.
- Once a flashback is seen, advance the catheter and needle by about 2 mm.
- Pull back slightly on the needle and advance the catheter into the vein. Alternatively, if the

catheter needle has a self-retracting needle, press the retracting button to retract the needle and then advance or 'hub' the catheter.
- Release the tourniquet.
- Press on the vein over the tip of the catheter, remove the needle completely (unless already removed as described above), and immediately put it into the sharps box.
- Cap the catheter. If drawing blood from the catheter, cap the catheter with a two-way cap, attach a vacuum tube adapter and fill blood bottles before flushing the line.
- Apply the adhesive plaster to fix the catheter.
- Flush the catheter with 5 ml normal saline.

Table 1. IV catheter sizes

Color	Size	Water flow (ml/min)*
Blue	22G	33
Pink	20G	54
Green	18G	80
	17G	125
Gray	16G	180
Orange	14G	270

* Approximate values. According to Poiseuille's Law, the velocity of a Newtonian fluid through a cylindrical tube is directly proportional to the fourth power of its radius.

After the procedure

- Discard any trash.
- Ensure that the patient is comfortable.
- Thank the patient.

Intravenous access and setting up a drip

The equipment

In a tray, gather:

- A pair of gloves.
- A tourniquet.
- Alcohol swabs.
- An IV catheter of appropriate size.
- Adhesive tape.
- A sharps box.
- An appropriate fluid bag.
- IV kit.

The procedure

- Check the fluid prescription chart (if appropriate).
- Check the fluid in the bag (solution type and concentration) and its expiry date.
- Remove the fluid bag from its packaging and hang it up on a drip stand.
- Remove the IV kit from its packaging. The regulating clamp for the IV line should be closed.
- Remove the protective covering from the exit port at the bottom end of the fluid bag.
- Remove the plastic cover from the large, pointed end of the IV kit.
- Drive the large, pointed end of the IV kit into the exit port at the bottom end of the fluid bag.
- Remove the protective cap from the other end of the IV kit.
- Squeeze and release the collecting chamber of the IV kit until it is about half full.

- Open the regulating clamp and run fluid through the IV kit to release any air/bubbles.
- Close the regulating clamp.
- Wash your hands (see *Station 1*).
- Position the patient so that his arm is fully extended. Ensure that he is comfortable.
- Apply the tourniquet.
- Select a vein by palpation: the bigger and straighter the better. Try to avoid the dorsum of the hand and the antecubital fossa.
- Don a pair of non-sterile gloves.
- Clean the skin with an alcohol swab and let it dry.
- Remove the IV catheter from its packaging and remove its cap.
- Tell the patient to expect a 'sharp scratch'.
- Anchor the vein by stretching the skin and insert the catheter at an angle of approximately 30 degrees.
- Once a flashback is seen, advance the catheter and needle by about 2 mm.
- Pull back slightly on the needle and advance the catheter into the vein.
- Release the tourniquet.
- Press on the vein over the tip of the catheter, remove the needle and immediately put it into the sharps box.
- Cap the catheter.

Indicate that you would:

- Apply the adhesive tape to secure the catheter.
- Attach the IV kit.
- Adjust the drip-rate (1 drop per second is equivalent to about 1 liter per 6 hours).
- Check that there is no swelling of the subcutaneous tissue.
- Tape the tubing to the arm.

After the procedure

- Ensure that the patient is comfortable.
- Thank the patient.
- Discard any trash.
- Sign the fluid chart and record the date and time (if appropriate).

Senior Resident's questions: complications of catheter insertion	
• Infiltration of the subcutaneous tissue	• Phlebitis
• Nerve damage	• Thrombophlebitis
• Hematoma	• Septic thrombophlebitis
• Embolism	• Local infection

Blood transfusion

While house officers do not usually set up a blood transfusion it is crucial to know the steps involved so that you can foresee any complications.

Before starting

- Introduce yourself to the patient.
- Explain the requirement for a blood transfusion and ensure that he is consenting.
- Ensure that vital signs have been recorded (pulse rate, blood pressure, and temperature).

Intravenous access

See *Station 4*.

Blood transfusion

1. Sample collection

- Confirm the patient's name and date of birth and check his identity bracelet.
- Extract 10 ml of blood into an appropriate type and screen tube.
- Immediately label the tube and request form with the patient's identifying data: name, date of birth, and hospital number.
- Fill out a blood transfusion form, specifying the total number of units required. If this process is performed electronically at your institution follow local procedures for ordering blood products.
- Ensure that the tube reaches the laboratory promptly.

2. Blood transfusion prescription

- Prescribe the number of units of blood required in the appropriate section of the patient's paper or electronic medical record. Each unit of blood should be prescribed separately and be administered over a period of 4 hours.
- If the patient is elderly or has a history of heart failure, and you are prescribing multiple units, consider also prescribing a diuretic to avoid volume overload.
- Arrange for the blood product to be delivered. The blood transfusion must start within 30 minutes of the blood leaving the blood refrigerator.

3. Checking procedures

Ask a registered nurse or another doctor to go through the following checking procedures with you:

- A. Positively identify the patient by asking him for his name, date of birth, and address.
- B. Confirm the patient's identifying data and ensure that they match those on his identity bracelet, case notes, medication record, and blood compatibility report.
- C. Record the blood group and serial number on the unit of blood and make sure that they match the blood group and serial number on the blood compatibility report and the blood compatibility label attached to the blood unit.
- D. Check the expiry date on the unit of blood.
- E. Inspect the blood bag for leaks or blood clots or discoloration.

4. Blood administration

- Attach one end of the transfusion giving set to the blood bag and run it through to ensure that any air in the tubing has been expelled. Note that a transfusion tubing set has an integral filter and is not the same as a standard fluid giving set.
- Attach the other end of the giving set to the IV catheter which should be a gray (16G), wide-bore catheter.
- Adjust the drip rate so that the unit of blood is administered over 4 hours. Because one unit of blood is 300 ml, and because 15 drops are equivalent to about 1 ml, this amounts to about 19 drops per minute.
- Sign the medication record and the blood compatibility report recording the date and time the transfusion was started. The medication record and blood compatibility report should also be signed by your checking co-worker.

5. Patient monitoring

- Record the patient's pulse rate, blood pressure, and temperature at 0, 15, and 30 minutes, and then hourly thereafter.
- Ensure that the nursing staff observe the patient for signs of adverse transfusion reactions such as fever, tachycardia, hypotension, urticaria, nausea, chest pain, and shortness of breath.
- Make an entry in the patient's notes, specifying the reason for the transfusion, the rate of the transfusion, the total number of units given, and any adverse transfusion reactions.

Senior Resident's questions: complications of blood transfusion	
Immune	• Acute hemolytic reaction, (usually due to ABO incompatibility)
	• Delayed hemolytic reaction, (usually due to Rhesus, Kell, Duffy, etc., incompatibility)
	• Non-hemolytic reactions such as febrile reactions, urticarial reactions, and anaphylaxis
Infectious	• Hepatitis
	• HIV/AIDS
	• Other viral agents
	• Bacteria
	• Parasites
Cardiovascular	• Left ventricular failure from volume overload
Complications of massive transfusion (>10 U)	• Hypothermia
	• Coagulopathy
	• Acid–base disturbances
	• Hyperkalemia
	• Citrate toxicity
	• Iron overload
Other	• Air embolism
	• Thrombophlebitis

Intramuscular, subcutaneous, and intradermal drug injection

Before starting

- Introduce yourself to the patient.
- Discuss the procedure and obtain consent.
- Ask the patient if he is allergic to the drug that is going to be injected.
- Gather the appropriate equipment.

The equipment

- Patient's drug chart.
- Drug.
- Dilutant (usually sterile water or saline).
- Appropriately sized syringe (e.g. 1 or 2 ml).
- 21G (green) needle and 23G (blue) or 25G (orange) needle*.

- Non-sterile gloves.
- Alcohol swab.
- Cotton swabs.
- Band-Aid.
- Sharps box.

*Note that the color scheme for needles is not the same as that for IV catheters (see *Station 4*)

The procedure

- Consult the medication record and check:
  - the identity of the patient
  - the prescription: validity, drug, dose, dilutant (if appropriate), route of administration, date and time of administration
  - drug allergies, anticoagulation
- Use your local formulary to check the form of the drug, whether it needs reconstituting, the type and volume of dilutant required, and the speed of administration.
- Check the name, dose and expiry date of the drug on the vial and ask another member of staff to double-check them.
- Wash your hands and don the gloves.
- Attach a 21G needle to the syringe and draw up the correct volume of the drug, making sure to tap out and expel any air. For a powder, inject the appropriate type and volume of dilutant into the ampoule and shake until the powder has dissolved.
- Remove the needle and attach a 23G needle to the syringe for IM/SC administration or a 25G needle for ID administration.
- Ask the patient to expose his upper arm or leg and ensure that the target muscle is completely relaxed.
- Identify landmarks in an attempt to avoid injuring nerves and vessels.
- Clean the exposed site with an alcohol swab and allow it to dry.

Intramuscular injection technique

- For older children and adults, the densest portion of the deltoid muscle (above the armpit and below the acromion) is the preferred IM injection site. The gluteal muscle is best avoided as the needle may not reach the muscle and there is a risk of damage to the sciatic nerve. In infants and toddlers, the vastus lateralis muscle in the anterolateral aspect of the middle or upper thigh is the preferred IM injection site.

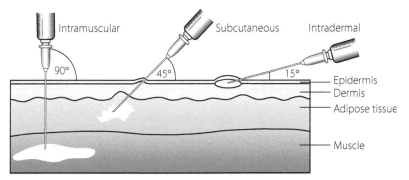

Figure 2. Intramuscular, subcutaneous, and intradermal injection techniques.

- With your free hand, slightly stretch the skin at the site of injection.
- Introduce the needle at an 80–90 degree angle to the patient's skin in a quick, firm motion.
- Pull on the syringe's plunger to ensure that you have not entered a blood vessel. If you aspirate blood, you need to start again with a new needle, and at a different site.
- Slowly inject the drug and quickly remove the needle.
- Immediately dispose of the needle in the sharps box.
- Apply gentle pressure over the injection site with a cotton swab.
- Remove the gloves.

Subcutaneous injection technique

- Bunch the skin between thumb and forefinger, thereby lifting the adipose tissue from the underlying muscle.
- Insert the needle at a 45 degree angle in a quick, firm motion.
- Release the skin.
- Pull on the syringe's plunger to ensure that you have not entered a blood vessel.
- Slowly inject the drug.
- Dispose of the needle in the sharps box.
- Apply gentle pressure over the injection site with a cotton swab.
- Remove the gloves.

Intradermal injection technique

- Stretch the skin taut between thumb and forefinger.
- Hold the needle so that the bevel is uppermost.
- Insert the needle at a 15 degree angle, almost parallel to the skin.
- Ensure that the needle is visible beneath the surface of the epidermis.
- Slowly inject the drug.
- A visible bleb should form. If not, immediately withdraw the needle and start again.
- Dispose of the needle in the sharps box.
- Remove the gloves.

After the procedure

- Ensure that the patient is comfortable.
- Sign the prescription chart and record the date, time, drug, dose, and injection site of the injection in the medical records.
- Ensure that the patient is comfortable.
- Ask him if he has any questions or concerns.
- Thank him.

Station 7

Blood pressure measurement

Before starting

- Introduce yourself to the patient.
- Explain the procedure and ask for his consent to carry it out.
- Tell him that he might feel some discomfort as the cuff is inflated, and that the blood pressure measurement may have to be repeated.

 Avoid white coat hypertension by putting the patient at ease. Briefly discuss a non-threatening subject, such as the patient's journey to the clinic, or the weather.

The procedure

- Select an appropriately sized cuff and attach it to the BP machine. This is usually a standard cuff in all but children and the obese.
- Position the patient's right arm so that it is horizontal at the level of the mid-sternum.
- Locate the brachial artery at about 2 cm above the antecubital fossa.
- Apply the cuff to the arm, ensuring that the arterial point is over the brachial artery.
- Inflate the cuff to 20–30 mmHg higher than the estimated systolic blood pressure. You can estimate the systolic blood pressure by palpating the brachial or radial artery pulse and inflating the cuff until you can no longer feel it.
- Place the stethoscope over the brachial artery pulse, ensuring that it does not touch the cuff.
- Reduce the pressure in the cuff at a rate of 2–3 mmHg.
  - The first consistent Korotkov sounds indicate the systolic blood pressure.
  - The muffling and disappearance of the Korotkov sounds indicate the diastolic blood pressure.
- Record the blood pressure as the systolic reading over the diastolic reading. Do not attempt to 'round off' your readings.
- If the blood pressure is higher than 140/90, indicate that you might take a second reading after giving the patient a one minute rest.
- In some situations, it may be appropriate to record the blood pressure in both arms, and also with the patient lying and standing.

After the procedure

- Ensure that the patient is comfortable.
- Tell the patient his blood pressure and explain its significance. Hypertension can only be confirmed by several blood pressure measurements taken over time or by home blood pressure measurement.
- Thank the patient.
- Document the blood pressure recording in the patient's notes.

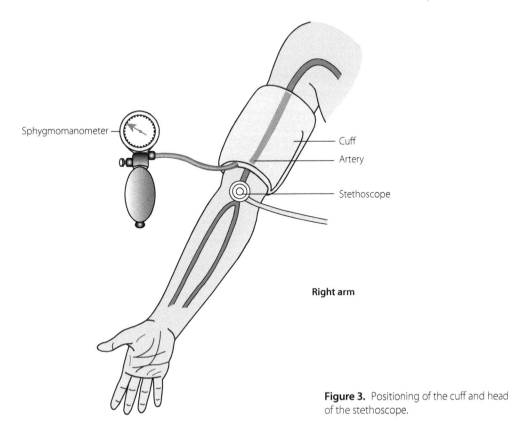

Sphygmomanometer

Cuff

Artery

Stethoscope

Right arm

Figure 3. Positioning of the cuff and head of the stethoscope.

Senior Resident's questions	
Causes of secondary hypertension:	**Complications of hypertension:**
• high catecholamines as in pheochromocytoma • high glucocorticoids as in Cushing's syndrome • high mineralocorticoids as in Conn's syndrome • renal disease • renal artery stenosis • coarctation of the aorta • hyper- or hypo-thyroidism • hyperparathyroidism • pre-eclampsia • illicit drugs	• cerebrovascular accident (hemorrhage or infarct) • retinopathy • ischemic heart disease • left ventricular failure • renal failure **Investigations in hypertension:** • this involves confirming hypertension, assessing for a possible secondary cause, and assessing for end-organ damage (see above)

Station 8

PEFR meter explanation

 Read in conjunction with Station 85: Explaining skills.

Before starting

- Introduce yourself to the patient.
- Check his understanding of asthma.
- Explain the importance of using a PEFR (Peak Expiratory Flow Rate) meter and the importance of using it correctly.
- Explain that the PEFR meter is to be used first thing in the morning and at any time he has symptoms of asthma.

Explain the use of a PEFR meter

Demonstrate and ask the patient to:

- Attach a clean mouthpiece to the meter.
- Slide the marker to the bottom of the numbered scale.
- Stand or sit up straight.
- Hold the peak flow meter horizontal, keeping his fingers away from the marker.
- Take as deep a breath as possible and hold it.
- Insert the mouthpiece into his mouth, sealing his lips around the mouthpiece.
- Exhale as hard as possible into the meter.
- Read and record the meter reading.
- Repeat the procedure three to six times, recording only the highest score.
- Check this score against the peak flow chart or his previous readings.
- Check the patient's understanding by asking him to carry out the procedure.

Ask him if he has any questions or concerns.

Interpret a PEFR reading

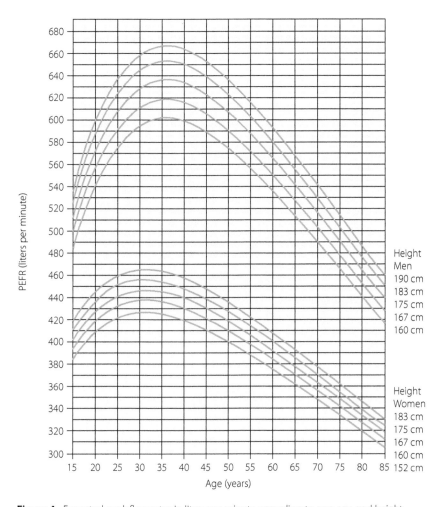

Figure 4. Expected peak flow rates in liters per minute according to age, sex, and height.

Clinical Skills for Medical Students

Station 9

Metered dose inhaler explanation

 Read in conjunction with Station 85: Explaining skills.

Before starting

- Introduce yourself to the patient.
- Check his understanding of asthma.
- Explain to him that an inhaler device delivers aerosolized bronchodilator medication for inhalation. If used correctly, it provides fast and efficient relief from bronchospasm (or airway irritation and narrowing). He can take up to two puffs from the inhaler, as required, up to four times a day. If he finds himself using the inhaler more frequently than this, then he should speak to his doctor. Possible side-effects of the bronchodilator medication are a fast heart rate, shakiness, and headaches.
- Ask him if he has any concerns.

Instruct on the use of an inhaler

Demonstrate and ask the patient to:

- Vigorously shake the inhaler.
- Remove the cap from the mouthpiece.
- Hold the inhaler between index finger and thumb.
- Place the inhaler upright about 3–5 cm in front of his mouth.
- Breathe out completely.
- Breathe in deeply, and simultaneously activate the inhaler.
- Close his mouth and hold his breath for 10 seconds and then breathe out.
- Repeat the procedure after 1 minute if relief is insufficient.
- Check his understanding by asking him to carry out the procedure.
- Ask him if he has any questions or concerns.

 If the patient has difficulty co-ordinating breathing in and inhaler activation, he may benefit from the added use of an aerochamber inhaler spacer.

Drug administration via a nebulizer

A nebulizer transforms a drug solution into a fine mist for inhalation via a mouthpiece or face mask. Drugs used in nebulizers include bronchodilators, corticosteroids, and antibiotics (e.g. colistin).

Before starting

- Introduce yourself to the patient.
- Explain the need for a nebulizer and the procedure involved, and ensure consent.
- Explain the drug in the nebulizer, most likely albuterol, and its common side-effects.
- Obtain consent.

The equipment

- An air compressor and tubing.
- A nebulizer cup.
- A mouthpiece or mask.
- A syringe.

- Drug or drug solution (e.g. albuterol 2.5 ml) in a vial.
- Dilutant (e.g. sodium chloride 0.9%) if needed.

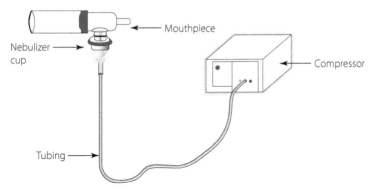

Figure 5. Nebulizer set-up.

The procedure

- Consult the prescription chart or electronic medical record and check:
  - the identity of the patient
  - the prescription: validity, drug, dose, dilutant, route of administration, date and time of starting
  - drug allergies
- Check the name, dose, and expiry date of the drug on the vial.
- Ask a co-worker (registered nurse or doctor) to confirm the name, dose, and expiry date of the drug on the vial.
- Place the air compressor on a sturdy surface and plug it into the wall power.

 As the compressor unit delivers a set airflow rate that is most suitable for asthmatic patients, it should not be used in COPD patients. For COPD patients, connect the tubing to the oxygen outlet in the wall and set the flow rate to 8 l/min.

- Wash your hands.
- Open the vial of drug solution by twisting off the top.
- With the syringe, carefully draw up the correct amount of drug solution.
- Remove the top part of the nebulizer cup and place the drug solution into it.
- Re-attach the top part of the nebulizer cup and connect the mouthpiece or face mask to the nebulizer cup.
- Connect the tubing from the air compressor to the bottom of the nebulizer cup.
- Switch on the air compressor and ensure that a fine mist is being produced.
- Ask the patient to sit up straight.
- If using a mouthpiece, ask him to clasp it between his teeth and to seal his lips around it. If using a mask, position it comfortably and securely over his face.
- Ask him to take slow, deep breaths through the mouth and, if possible, to hold each breath for 2–3 seconds before breathing out.
- Continue until there is no drug left and the nebulizer begins to splutter (about 10 minutes).
- Turn the compressor off.
- Ask the patient to take several deep breaths and to cough up any secretions.
- Ask him to rinse his mouth with water.
- Wash your hands.
- Sign the prescription chart, if applicable.

 Should the patient feel dizzy, he should interrupt the treatment and rest for about 5 minutes. After resuming the treatment, he should be instructed to breathe more slowly through the mouthpiece.

After the procedure

- Clean and disinfect the equipment.
- Sign the drug chart and record the dilutant used, and the date, time, and dose of the drug in the medical records or in the electronic medical record.
- Indicate that you would have your checking co-worker countersign it.
- Ask the patient if he has any questions or concerns.
- Ensure that he is comfortable.

Nasogastric intubation

Specifications: A mannequin in lieu of a patient.

Choice of NG tube

Nasogastric (NG or Ryle's) tubes can be used for feeding or drug administration, to decompress the stomach, to obtain a sample of gastric fluid, or to drain the stomach's contents (e.g. after an overdose or if emergency surgery is required). If the tube is being used for aspiration or drainage, a gauge of 10 or greater is required. If not, a fine bore tube should be preferred.

The equipment

- A pair of non-sterile gloves.
- An NG tube of appropriate size.
- Water-soluble lubricant.
- Topical anesthetic spray.
- A glass of water with a straw.
- Tape.
- Stethoscope.
- A 20 ml syringe and some pH paper.
- A spigot or catheter bag.
- An emesis basin.

Before starting

- Introduce yourself to the patient.
- Explain the need for an NG tube and the procedure for inserting it, and ensure consent.
- Position the patient upright and ask about nostril preference/examine the nostrils.
- Ensure that the patient is comfortable.

The procedure

- Gather the equipment.
- Wash your hands and don the gloves.
- Measure the length of NG tube to be inserted by placing the tip of the tube at the nostril and extending the tube behind the ear and then to two fingerbreadths above the umbilicus.
- Lubricate the tip of the NG tube with water-soluble lubricant.
- Spray the back of the throat with topical anesthetic or state that you would do so.
- Insert the NG tube into the preferred nostril and slide it along the floor of the nose into the nasopharynx.
- Ask the patient to tilt his head forward and to swallow some water through a straw as you continue to advance the tube through the pharynx and esophagus and into the stomach. Each time the patient swallows, advance the tube a little bit further.
- If the patient coughs or gags, slightly withdraw the tube and leave him some time to recover.
- Insert the tube to the required length.
- Ensure that the tip of the tube is in the stomach.
  - Inject 20 ml of air into the tube and listen over the epigastrium with your stethoscope.
  - Pull back on the plunger to aspirate stomach contents. Test the aspirate with pH paper to confirm its acidity (pH < 6). If a fine-bore tube has been inserted, it may not be possible to aspirate stomach contents.
  - Request a chest X-ray or indicate that you would do so, as neither of the aforementioned techniques can reliably confirm NG tube placement.
- Tape the tube to the nose and to the side of the face.
- Attach a spigot or catheter bag to the NG tube.

Clinical Skills for Medical Students

After the procedure

- Ask the patient if he has any questions or concerns.
- Ensure that he is comfortable.
- Thank him.
- Make an entry in the patient's medical record.

[Note]   The principal complications of NG tube insertion are aspiration and tissue trauma.

Male catheterization

Specifications: A male anatomical model in lieu of a patient.

Before starting

- Introduce yourself to the patient.
- Explain the procedure and ask for his consent to carry it out.
- Position him flat on the exam table with legs apart and groin exposed.

The equipment
On a clean tray, gather:

- A catheterization pack.
- Saline solution.
- Sterile gloves.
- A 10 ml pre-filled syringe containing 2% lidocaine gel.
- A 12–16 french Foley catheter.
- A catheter bag.
- A 10 ml syringe containing sterile water.
- Adhesive tape.

The procedure

- Gather the equipment.
- Check the expiry date of the catheter.
- Open the catheter pack aseptically onto a tray, attach the yellow bag to the side of the tray, and pour saline solution into the receiver.
- If pre-filled syringes are not provided with the pack, draw up 10 ml sterile water and 10 ml lidocaine gel into separate syringes.
- Wash and dry your hands.
- Put on sterile gloves.
- Drape the patient.
- Place a collecting vessel between the patient's legs.
- With your non-dominant hand, hold the penis with a sterile swab.
- With your dominant hand, retract the foreskin, if present, and clean the area around the urethral meatus with saline-soaked swabs. So as not to break sterility, hold the swabs with plastic prongs, and use one set of prongs per swab.
- Coat the end of the catheter with lidocaine gel and instil 10 ml of lidocaine gel into the urethra. Hold the urethral meatus closed.
- Indicate that the anesthetic needs about 5 minutes to work.
- Hold the penis so that it is vertical.
- Holding the catheter by its sleeve, gently and progressively insert it into the urethra. Upon feeling resistance from the prostate, hold the penis horizontally so as to facilitate insertion.
- Once a stream of urine is obtained, inject 10 ml of sterile water to inflate the catheter's balloon, continually ensuring that this does not cause the patient any pain.
- Gently retract the catheter until a resistance is felt.
- Attach the catheter bag.
- Reposition the foreskin.
- Tape the catheter to the thigh.

After the procedure

- Ensure that the patient is comfortable.
- Thank the patient.
- Discard any trash.
- Record the date and time of catheterization, type and size of catheter used, volume of water used to inflate the balloon, and volume of urine in the catheter bag.

Senior Resident's questions

Indications for catheterization:

- hygienic care of bedridden patients
- monitoring of urine output
- acute urinary retention
- chronic obstruction
- collection of a specimen of uncontaminated urine
- irrigation of the bladder
- imaging of the urinary tract

Contraindications:

- pelvic trauma
- previous stricture
- previous failure to catheterize
- severe phimosis

Complications:

- paraphimosis (from failure to reposition the foreskin)
- urethral perforation and creation of false passages
- bleeding
- infection
- urethral strictures

Female catheterization

Specifications: A female anatomical model in lieu of a patient.

Before starting

- Introduce yourself to the patient.
- Explain the procedure and ask for her consent to carry it out.
- Ask her to undress from the waist down and place a sheet over her.

The equipment
On a clean tray, gather:

- Two pairs of sterile gloves.
- A catheterization pack.
- Saline solution.
- A 12–16 french Foley catheter.
- A 10 ml pre-filled syringe containing 2% lidocaine gel.
- A 10 ml syringe containing sterile water.
- A catheter bag.
- Adhesive tape.

The procedure

- Gather the equipment.
- Open the catheter pack aseptically onto a tray, attach the yellow bag to the side of the tray, and pour antiseptic solution into the receiver.
- If pre-filled syringes are not provided with the pack, draw up 10 ml sterile water and 10 ml lidocaine into separate syringes.
- Wash and dry your hands.
- Put on both pairs of gloves (practice this – it's not easy).
- Ask the patient to remove her sheet and lie flat on the exam table, bringing her heels to her buttocks and then letting her knees flop out.
- Drape the patient.
- Place a collecting vessel between the patient's legs.
- Use your non-dominant hand to separate the labia minora.
- Clean the area around the urethral meatus with saline-soaked swabs.
- Coat the end of the catheter with lidocaine gel and instil 5 ml of lidocaine into the urethra.
- Indicate that the anesthetic needs about 5 minutes to work.
- Discard the outer pair of gloves.
- Holding the catheter by its sleeve, gently and progressively insert it into the urethra.
- Once a stream of urine is obtained, inject 10 ml of sterile water to inflate the catheter's balloon, continually ensuring that this does not cause the patient any pain.
- Gently retract the catheter until a resistance is felt.
- Attach the catheter bag.
- Tape the catheter to the thigh.

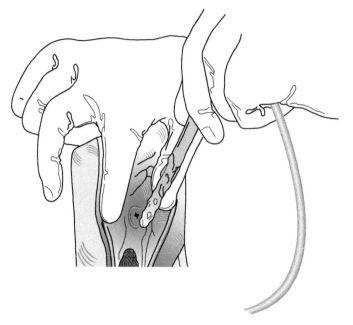

Figure 6. Preparing to insert the catheter.

After the procedure

- Ensure that the patient is comfortable.
- Thank the patient.
- Discard any trash.
- Record the date and time of catheterization, type and size of catheter used, volume of water used to inflate the balloon, and volume of urine in the catheter bag.

Wound suturing

General skills and procedures

Specifications: In an exam you may be provided with a pad of 'skin' in lieu of a patient. This station most likely requires you to talk through the parts of the procedure and then to demonstrate your suturing technique. For this second part, there can be no substitute for practice, practice, and more practice!

Before starting

- Introduce yourself to the patient.
- Explain the procedure and ask for his consent to carry it out.
- Examine the wound, looking for debris, dirt, and tendon damage.
- Indicate that you would request an X-ray to exclude a foreign body.
- Assess distal motor, sensory, and vascular function.
- Position the patient appropriately and ensure that he is comfortable.

The equipment

Gather in a tray:

- a pair of sterile gloves
- a suture pack
- a suture of appropriate type (monofilament non-absorbable for superficial wounds, absorbable for deep wounds) and size (3/0 for scalp and trunk, 4/0 for limbs, 5/0 for hands, 6/0 for face)
- a 5 ml syringe, 21G and 25G needles, and a vial of local anesthetic (e.g. 1% lidocaine)
- antiseptic solution
- a sharps bin

The procedure

- Wash your hands.
- Open the suture pack, thus creating a sterile field.
- Pour antiseptic solution into the receptacle.
- Open the suture, the syringe, and both needles onto the sterile field.
- Wash your hands using sterile technique.
- Don the non-sterile gloves.
- Attach a 21G needle to the syringe.
- Ask an assistant (the examiner) to open the vial of local anesthetic and draw up 5 ml of local anesthetic. For an average 70 kg adult, up to 20 ml of 1% lidocaine can be safely used, although 5–10 ml is usually sufficient. Epinephrine may be used with lidocaine to minimize bleeding. The maximum safe dose of lidocaine with or without epinephrine is 7 mg/kg and 3 mg/kg respectively. However, avoid injecting epinephrine when anesthetizing the extremities due to the risk of ischemic tissue necrosis.
- Discard the needle into the sharps bin and attach the 25G needle to the syringe.
- Clean the wound (use forceps) with a cotton swab soaked in antiseptic and drape the field. Dirty wounds may benefit from cleansing with povidone iodine, whereas normal saline can be used to cleanse and irrigate 'clean' wounds.
- Inject the local anesthetic into the apices and edges of the wound. Make sure to pull back on the plunger before injecting.
- Discard the needle into the sharps bin.
- Indicate that you would give the anesthetic 5–10 minutes to operate (or as long as it takes).

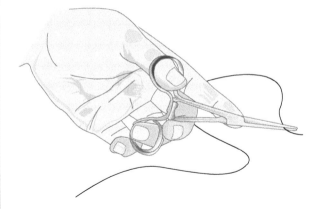

Figure 7. Use needle-holding forceps to hold the needle approximately two-thirds from the needle tip.

- Apply the sutures approximately 3 mm from the wound edge and 5–10 mm apart. Use needle-holding forceps to hold the needle and toothed forceps to pick up the skin margins. Knot the sutures around the needle-holding forceps.

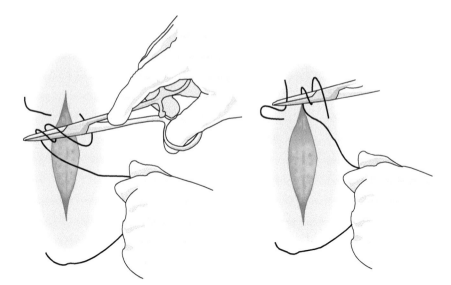

Figure 8. Suggested approach for suturing. Knot the sutures around the needle-holding forceps: loop the suture twice around the nose of the needle-holding forceps using your hand. Then take hold of the short end of the suture with the needle-holding forceps and carry it through the loops, gently pulling the knot tight. Two further single loops are then added in a similar fashion to secure the knot. Each loop is pulled in the opposite direction across the wound edge.

After the procedure

- Clean the wound and indicate that you would apply a dressing.
- Assess the need for a tetanus injection.
- Give appropriate instructions for wound care and indicate the date sutures should be removed (e.g. face 3–4 days, scalp 5 days, trunk 7 days, limbs 7–10 days, feet 10–14 days).
- Ask if the patient has any questions or concerns.
- Thank the patient.

Chest pain history

Before starting

- Introduce yourself to the patient.
- Explain that you are going to ask him some questions to uncover the nature of his chest pain, and ask for his consent to do this.
- Ensure that he is comfortable; if not, make sure that he is.

The history

- Name, age, occupation, and ethnic origin.

Chief complaint and history of chief complaint

First use open questions to get the patient's history, including any previous episodes of chest pain, and elicit his ideas, concerns, and expectations. Give the patient time to tell his story, and remember to be empathetic: chest pain can be a very frightening experience.

Then ask specifically about:

- **S**ite. Ask the patient to point to the site of the pain.
- **O**nset and progression.
- **C**haracter.
- **R**adiation (into the jaw, arm, or back).
- **A**ssociated symptoms and signs.
  - Sweating.
  - Nausea and vomiting.
  - Shortness of breath.
  - Dizziness.
  - Cough.
  - Hemoptysis.
  - Palpitations.
- **T**iming and duration.
- **E**xacerbating and relieving factors; for example, exercise, movement, deep breathing, coughing, cold air, large or spicy meals, alcohol, rest, TNG, sitting up in bed.
- **S**everity. Ask the patient to rate the pain on a scale of 1 to 10, with 1 being no pain at all, and 10 being the worst pain they have ever experienced. Determine the effect that it is having on his everyday life, including exercise tolerance and sleep.

Socrates (470–399 BC)

Whither haste ye, O men? Yea, verily ye know not that ye are doing none of the things ye ought …

Past medical history

- Current, past, and childhood illnesses.
- In particular, ask about coronary heart disease, myocardial infarction, stroke, pneumonia, pulmonary embolism, deep vein thrombosis, hypertension, hyperlipidemia, diabetes, smoking, alcohol use, history of gastroesophageal reflux disease and recent long-haul travel.
- Recent trauma or injury.
- Surgery.

Drug history

- Prescribed medication, including the oral contraceptive pill if female.
- Over-the-counter medication.
- Illicit drugs, especially cocaine.
- Allergies.

Family history

- Parents, siblings, and children. Ask specifically about heart disease, hypertension, and other heritable cardiovascular risk factors, also history of sudden death.

Social history

- Employment.
- Housing.
- Hobbies.

After taking the history

- Ask the patient if there is anything else that he might add that you have forgotten to ask. This is an excellent question to ask in clinical practice, and an even better one to ask in exams.
- Thank the patient.
- Summarize your findings and consider a differential diagnosis.
- State that you would like to examine the patient and order some investigations, for example, ECG and chest X-ray, to confirm your diagnosis.

MI: the evidence	
For MI	**Against MI**
• Chest pain radiating to both arms (positive LR, 7.1) • 3rd heart sound (positive LR, 3.2) • Hypotension (positive LR, 3.1)	• Pleuritic chest pain (negative LR, 0.2) • Chest pain reproduced by palpation (negative LR, 0.2–0.4) • Sharp or stabbing chest pain (negative LR, 0.2)
LR = likelihood ratio. For a full discussion of likelihood ratios see the Appendix. [*JAMA* (1988), **280**: 1256–1263]	

Common conditions most likely to come up in a chest pain history station
Angina: • heavy retrosternal pain which may radiate into the neck or left arm • brought on by effort and relieved by rest and nitrates • risk factors for ischemic heart disease are likely • a family history of ischemic heart disease is likely

Cardiovascular and respiratory medicine

MI:
- pain typically comes on over a few minutes
- pain is similar to that of angina but is typically severe, long-lasting (> 20 minutes), and unresponsive to nitrates
- often associated with sweating, nausea, and shortness of breath
- risk factors for ischemic heart disease are likely
- a family history of ischemic heart disease is likely

Pleuritic pain:
- sharp, stabbing, 'catching' pain
- may radiate to the back or shoulder
- typically aggravated by deep breathing and coughing
- can be caused by pleurisy which can occur with pneumonia, pulmonary embolus, and pneumothorax, or by pericarditis which can occur post-MI, in viral infections, and in autoimmune diseases
- pleural pain is localized to one side of the chest and is not position dependent
- pericardial pain is central and positional, aggravated by lying down and alleviated by sitting up or leaning forward

Pulmonary embolus:
- sharp, stabbing pain that is of sudden onset
- may be associated with shortness of breath, hemoptysis, and/or pleurisy
- typically aggravated by deep breathing and coughing
- risk factors such as recent surgery or prolonged bed rest may be present

Gastroesophageal reflux disease:
- retrosternal burning
- clear relationship with food and alcohol, but no relationship with effort
- may be associated with odynophagia and nocturnal asthma
- aggravated by lying down and alleviated by sitting up and by antacids such as Pepto-Bismol or milk

Musculoskeletal complaint:
- may be associated with a history of physical injury or unusual exertion
- pain is aggravated by movement, but is not reliably alleviated by rest
- the site of the pain is tender to touch

Panic attack:
- rapid onset of severe anxiety lasting for about 20–30 minutes
- associated with chest tightness and hyperventilation

 If you cannot differentiate angina from gastroesophageal reflux disease, advise a therapeutic trial of an antacid and/or record an ECG.

Station 16

Cardiovascular risk assessment

Cardiovascular risk factors can usefully be divided into fixed (non-modifiable) and modifiable risk factors. Fixed risk factors include older age, male gender, family history, and a South Asian background. Modifiable risk factors include hypertension, hyperlipidemia, diabetes, smoking, alcohol, exercise, and stress. Having one or more of these risk factors does not mean that a person is going to develop cardiovascular disease, but merely that he is at increased probability of developing it. Conversely, having no risk factors is not a guarantee that a person is not going to develop cardiovascular disease.

Before starting

- Introduce yourself to the patient.
- Explain that you are going to ask him some questions to assess his risk of cardiovascular disease (coronary heart disease, cerebrovascular disease, vascular disease) and ask for his consent to do this.

 Remember to be tactful in your questioning, and to respond sensitively to the patient's ideas and concerns.

The risk assessment

If this information has not already been provided or disclosed, find out the patient's reason for presenting to the clinic or hospital. Then note or enquire about:

Fixed risk factors

1. Age.
2. Sex.
3. Ethnic background. People from a South Asian background are at a notably higher risk of cardiovascular disease.
4. Family history. Ask about a family history of cardiovascular disease and risk factors for cardiovascular disease such as hypertension, hyperlipidemia and diabetes mellitus.

Modifiable risk factors

5. Hypertension. If hypertensive, ask about latest blood pressure measurement, time since first diagnosis, and any medication being taken.
6. Hyperlipidemia. If hyperlipidemic, ask about latest serum cholesterol level, time since first diagnosis, and any medication being taken.
7. Diabetes mellitus. If diabetic, ask about medication being taken, level of diabetes control being achieved, time since first diagnosis, and presence of complications.
8. Cigarette smoking. If a smoker or ex-smoker, ask about number of years spent smoking and average number of cigarettes smoked per day. Does the patient also smoke hand-rolled cigarettes and/or cannabis?
9. Alcohol. Ask about the amount of alcohol drunk in a day. Note that depending on the amount and type that is drunk, alcohol can be either a protective factor or a risk factor.
10. Lack of exercise. Ask about amount of exercise taken in a day or week. Does the patient walk to work or walk to the shops?
11. Stress. Ask about occupational history and home life.

Table 2. Desirable lipid levels	
Total cholesterol	≤ 200 mg/dL
LDL cholesterol (fasting)	< 130 mg/dL
HDL cholesterol	≥ 60 mg/dL
Total cholesterol/HDL cholesterol	≤ 4.5
Tryglycerides (fasting)	≤ 150 mg/dL

NB. Patients at high risk of cardiovascular disease should aim
for even better than these figures.

After the assessment

- If you have time, assess the extent of any cardiovascular disease.
- Ask the patient if there is anything he would like to add that you may have forgotten to ask about.
- Consider using a validated cardiovascular risk calculator such as the Framingham Coronary Heart Disease Risk Score to determine 10-year risk; available free online.
- Give him feedback on his cardiovascular risk (e.g. low, medium, high), and indicate a further course of action if appropriate (e.g. further investigations or further appointment to discuss reducing modifiable risk factors).
- Address any remaining concerns.

Cardiovascular examination

Before starting

- Introduce yourself to the patient.
- Explain the examination and ask for his consent to carry it out.
- Position him at 45 degrees, and ask him to remove his top(s).
- Ensure that he is comfortable.

The examination

General inspection

- From the end of the exam table, observe the patient's general appearance (age, state of health, nutritional status, and any other obvious signs). Is he short of breath or cyanosed? Is he coughing? Does he have the malar flush of mitral stenosis?
- Observe the patient's surroundings, looking in particular for items such as a nitrate spray, an oxygen mask, and IV lines and infusions.
- Inspect the chest for any scars and the precordium for any abnormal pulsation. A median sternotomy scar could indicate coronary artery bypass grafting (CABG), valve repair or replacement, or the repair of a congenital defect. A left submammary scar most likely indicates repair or replacement of the mitral valve. Do not miss a pacemaker if it is there!

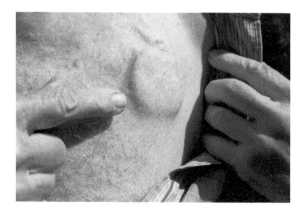

Figure 9. Pacemakers can be visible from outside the body.

Reproduced with permission from Julia Freeman-Woolpert (www.sxc.hu/profile/julia).

Inspection and examination of the hands

- Take both hands noting:
  - temperature. N.B. Determining whether the patient appears to have adequate cardiac output (is 'warm') or poor cardiac output (is 'cold') is a crucial part of managing patients with heart failure (see *JAMA* (2002) **287**: 628).
  - color (the blue of peripheral cyanosis and the orange of nicotine stains)
  - nail bed capillary refill time
  - the presence of clubbing (endocarditis, cyanotic congenital heart disease)
  - the presence of Osler nodes and Janeway lesions (subacute infective endocarditis (see *Figure 10*))
  - the presence of splinter hemorrhages (subacute infective endocarditis)
  - the presence of koilonychia or 'spoon nails' (iron deficiency)
- Determine the rate, rhythm, volume, and character of the radial pulse.

- Raise the patient's arm above his head to assess for a collapsing or water hammer pulse (aortic regurgitation). Ask the patient whether he has any shoulder pain first.
- Simultaneously take the pulse in both arms to exclude radio-radial delay (aortic arch aneurysm). Indicate that you would also exclude radio-femoral delay (coarctation of the aorta).
- As you move up the arm, look for bruising, which may indicate that the patient is on an anti-coagulant, and for evidence of intravenous drug use, which is a risk factor for subacute infective endocarditis.
- Indicate that you would like to record the blood pressure (see *Station 7*).

Pulsus paradoxus

This describes the exaggerated variation in blood pressure with inspiration (≥ 10 mm Hg) seen in conditions such as cardiac tamponade, constrictive pericarditis, and COPD. Literally, it refers to the paradox that a peripheral pulse may be absent in the present of audible heart sounds.

How to measure a pulsus paradoxus

- Inflate the cuff to obscure the Korotkoff sounds completely.
- Gradually deflate the cuff until the first Korotkoff sound is audible only in expiration, and record the systolic BP.
- Deflate the cuff until the Korotkoff sounds are heard continuously, i.e. during both expiration and inspiration, and record the systolic BP.
- Measure the difference in systolic BP. If ≥ 10 pulsus paradoxus is likely to be present.

Cardiac tamponade: the evidence	
For cardiac tamponade	**Against cardiac tamponade**
• A pulsus paradoxus of greater than 10 mm Hg (Positive LR 3.3)	• A pulsus paradoxus of less than 10 mm HG (Negative LR 0.03)
[*JAMA* (2007), **297**: 1810–1818]	

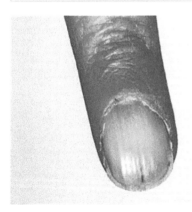

Figure 10. Splinter hemorrhage.

Inspection and examination of the head and neck

- Inspect the eyes, looking for peri-orbital xanthelasma and corneal arcus, both of which indicate hyperlipidemia.
- Gently retract an eyelid and ask the patient to look up. Inspect the conjunctivus for pallor, which is indicative of anemia.
- Ask the patient to open his mouth, and look for signs of central cyanosis, dehydration, poor dental hygiene (subacute bacterial endocarditis), and a high arched palate (Marfan's syndrome).
- Palpate the carotid artery and assess its volume and character. Never palpate both carotid arteries simultaneously.

- Assess the jugular venous pressure (see *Figure 11*) and, if possible, the jugular venous pulse form: ask the patient to turn his head slightly to one side, and look at the internal vein medial to the clavicular head of sternocleidomastoid. Assuming that the patient is reclining at 45 degrees, the vertical height of the jugular distension from the angle of Louis (sternal angle) should be no greater than 4 cm.

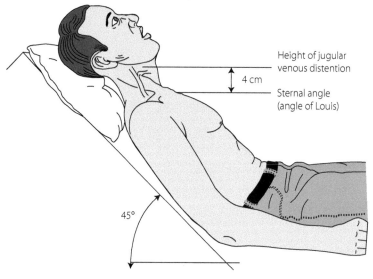

Height of jugular venous distention

4 cm

Sternal angle (angle of Louis)

45°

Figure 11. Assessing the jugular venous pressure.

Palpation of the heart

 Ask the patient if he has any chest pain.

- Determine the location and character of the apex beat. It is normally located in the fifth intercostal space at the midclavicular line. The apex may be displaced, and it may be 'heaving', suggesting left ventricular hypertrophy, or 'tapping', suggesting mitral stenosis.
- Place the flat of your hands over either side of the sternum and feel for any heaves and thrills. Heaves result from right ventricular hypertrophy (*cor pulmonale*) and thrills result from transmitted murmurs.

Heart failure: the evidence	
For heart failure	**Against heart failure**
• The presence of an S3 (LR of 11)	• The absence of rales/crackles (negative LR 0.51)
[*JAMA* (2005), **294**: 1944–1956]	

Auscultation of the heart

- Listen for heart sounds, additional sounds, murmurs, and pericardial rub. Using the stethoscope's diaphragm, listen in the:
  - *aortic area*
    right second intercostal space near the sternum
  - *pulmonary area*
    left second intercostal space near the sternum
  - *tricuspid area*
    left third, fourth, and fifth intercostal spaces near the sternum
  - *mitral area*
    left fifth intercostal space, in the mid-clavicular line

Auscultation points

Mid-clavicular
line

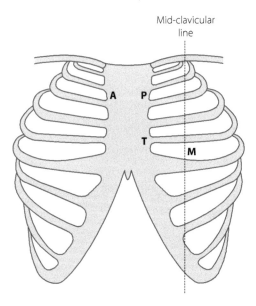

Figure 12. Auscultation points.

- In addition:
  - ask the patient to bend forward and to hold his breath at end-expiration. Using the stetho-scope's diaphragm, listen at the left sternal edge in the fourth intercostal space for the early to mid-diastolic murmur of aortic regurgitation.
  - ask the patient to turn onto his left side and to hold his breath at end-expiration. Using the stethoscope's *bell*, listen in the mitral area for the mid-diastolic murmur of mitral stenosis.
  - listen over the carotid arteries for any bruits and the radiation of the murmur of aortic stenosis.
  - listen in the left axilla for the radiation of the murmur of mitral regurgitation.

For any murmur, determine its location and radiation, and its duration and timing in relation to the cardiac cycle. This is best done by palpating the carotid artery to determine the start of systole. Grade the murmur on a scale of I to VI according to its intensity (see *Table 3*). Common conditions associated with murmurs are listed in *Table 4*.

Aortic regurgitation: the evidence
For at least mild aortic regurgitation • An early diastolic murmur (Positive LR 8.8–32)
[*JAMA* (1999), **281**: 2231–2238]

Table 3.	Grading murmurs
I	Barely audible
II	Soft but easily heard
III	Loud without a thrill
IV	Loud with a thrill
V	Loud with minimal contact of stethoscope to chest
VI	Audible without stethoscope

Table 4. Common conditions associated with murmurs	
Aortic stenosis	Slow-rising pulse, heaving cardiac apex, mid-systolic murmur best heard in the aortic area and radiating to the carotids and cardiac apex
Mitral regurgitation	Displaced, thrusting cardiac apex, pan-systolic murmur best heard in the mitral area and radiating to the axilla
Aortic regurgitation	Collapsing pulse, thrusting cardiac apex, diastolic murmur best heard at the left sternal edge
Mitral valve prolapse	Mid-systolic click, late-systolic murmur best heard in the mitral area

Chest examination

- Percuss and auscultate the chest, especially at the bases of the lungs. Heart failure can cause pulmonary edema and pleural effusions.

Abdominal examination

- Palpate the abdomen to exclude ascites and/or hepatomegaly.
- Check for the presence of an aortic aneurysm.
- Ballot the kidneys and listen for any renal artery bruits.

Examination of the ankles and legs

- Inspect the legs for scars that might be indicative of vein harvesting for a CABG.
- Palpate for the 'pitting' edema of cardiac failure, which in some cases may extend all the way up to the sacrum or even the torso ('anasarca').
- Assess the temperature of the feet, and check the posterior tibial and dorsalis pedis pulses in both feet.

After the examination

- Indicate that you would look at the observation chart, dipstick the urine, examine the retina with an ophthalmoscope and, if appropriate, order some key investigations, e.g. CBC, serum B-type naturiuretic peptide, ECG, CXR, echocardiogram.
- Cover the patient up and ensure that he is comfortable.
- Thank the patient.
- Summarize your findings and offer a differential diagnosis.

Common conditions most likely to come up in a cardiovascular examination station

- Murmurs (see *Table 4*)
- Heart failure
- Median sternotomy scar
- Pacemaker

Peripheral vascular system examination

This involves examination of both the arterial and venous systems. An integrated approach is presented below, which most closely mirrors that used in everyday practice.

Before starting

- Introduce yourself to the patient.
- Explain the examination and ask for his consent to carry it out.
- Ask him to expose his feet and legs and to lie down on the exam table.

The examination

Inspection

- Skin changes: pallor, shininess, loss of body hair, *atrophie blanche* (ivory-white areas), hemosiderin pigmentation, inflammation, eczema, lipodermatosclerosis.
- Thickened dystrophic nails.
- Scars.
- Signs of gangrene: blackened skin, nail infection, amputated toes.
- Venous and arterial ulcers. Remember to look in the interdigital spaces.
- Edema.
- Varicose veins (ask the patient to stand up). Varicose veins are often associated with incompetent valves in the long and short saphenous veins.

 Do not make the common mistake of asking the patient to stand up before having examined for varicose veins.

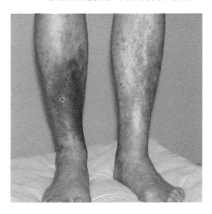

Figure 13. Lipodermatosclerosis describes areas of induration resulting from fibrosis of the subcutaneous fat, and may complicate chronic venous insufficiency.
Reproduced from www.surgicalnotes.co.uk.

Peripheral artery disease: the evidence

For peripheral artery disease in symptomatic patients
- Presence of claudication (positive LR 3.3)
- Cool skin (positive LR 5.9)
- Palpable pulse abnormality (positive LR 4.7)
- Presence of at least 1 bruit (positive LR 5.6)

[*JAMA* (2006), **295**: 536–546]

Clinical Skills for Medical Students

Palpation and special tests

- Ask about any pain in the legs and feet.
- Assess skin temperature by running the back of your hand along the leg and the sole of the foot. Compare both legs.
- Capillary refill. Compress a nail bed for 5 seconds and let go. It should take less than 2 seconds for the nail bed to return to its normal color.
  - Peripheral pulses (compare both sides).
  - Femoral pulse at the inguinal ligament.
  - Popliteal pulse in the popliteal space (flex the knee).
  - Posterior tibial pulse behind the medial malleolus.
  - *Dorsalis pedis* pulse over the dorsum of the foot, just lateral to the extensor tendon of the big toe.
- Buerger's test:
  - lift both of the patient's legs to a 15 degree angle and note any collapse of the veins ('venous guttering'), which is indicative of arterial insufficiency
  - lift both of the patient's legs up to the point where they turn white (this is Buerger's angle); if there is no arterial insufficiency, the legs will not turn white, not even at a 90 degree angle
  - ask the patient to dangle his legs over the edge of the exam table; in chronic limb ischemia, rather than returning to its normal color, the skin will slowly turn red like a cooked lobster (reactive hyperemia)
- Edema. Firm 'non-pitting' edema is a sign of chronic venous insufficiency (compare to the 'pitting' edema of cardiac failure).
- Varicose veins. Tenderness on palpation suggests thrombophlebitis.
- Trendelenburg's test:
  - elevate the leg to 90 degrees to drain the veins of blood
  - occlude the sapheno-femoral junction (SFJ) with two fingers
  - keep your fingers in place and ask the patient to stand up
  - remove your fingers: if the superficial veins refill, this indicates incompetence at the SFJ
- Tourniquet test:
  - elevate the leg to 90 degrees to drain the veins of blood
  - apply a tourniquet to the upper thigh
  - ask the patient to stand up: if the superficial veins below the tourniquet refill, this indicates incompetent perforators below the tourniquet
  - release the tourniquet: sudden additional filling of the veins is a sign of sapheno-femoral incompetence

[Note] The tourniquet test can be repeated further and further down the leg, until the superficial veins below the tourniquet no longer refill.

Auscultation

- Femoral arteries.
- Abdominal aorta.

After the examination

- Thank the patient.
- Ensure that he is comfortable.
- Summarize your findings and offer a differential diagnosis.
- If appropriate, indicate that you might also measure the ABPI and examine the cardiovascular system and abdomen (aortic aneurysm).

Table 5. Examination of the arterial or venous system only

Arterial system	Venous system
Pallor	*Atrophie blanche*
Shininess	Pigmentation
Dystrophic nails	Inflammation
Loss of body hair	Eczema
Arterial ulcers	Lipodermatosclerosis
Signs of gangrene	Edema (non-pitting)
Skin temperature	Venous ulcers
Capillary refill	Varicose veins
Peripheral pulses	Scars due to varicose vein surgery
Buerger's test	Trendelenburg test
Auscultation of femoral arteries and aorta	Perthes' test
ABPI (if time permits, see *Station 20*)	

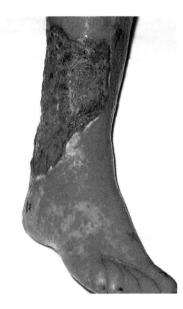

Figure 14. Large venous ulcer. Arterial and neuropathic ulcers tend to be on the sole of the foot and on pressure points, and venous ulcers on the medial and lateral aspects of the leg, above the malleoli.

Reproduced from *BMJ* (2000) **320:** 1589–91, with permission.

Cardiovascular and respiratory medicine

Station 19

Volume status examination

This station should be read in conjunction with *Stations 17* and *18*.

The assessment of a patient's volume status is a vital part of routine clinical assessment and determining whether the patient is euvolemic, hypervolemic, or hypovolemic is frequently an important branch point in clinical decision-making. This examination focuses on features that provide the most information about volume status.

Before starting

- Introduce yourself to the patient.
- Explain the examination and ask for his consent to carry it out.
- Position him at 45 degrees and expose the peripheries.

Hypovolemia: the evidence
The positive and negative LR for each finding predicting hypovolemia not due to blood loss, specifically, are given in parentheses.
[*JAMA* (1999), **11**: 1022–1029]

The examination

General inspection

- Confusion (positive LR 2.1) or unclear speech (positive LR 3.1) can be associated with dehydration.

Hands

- Delayed capillary refill time (normal at air temp of 21°C or 70°F: 2 sec for children and adult men, 3 sec for women; 4 sec for elderly [≥ 62 years old]) (Positive LR 6.9).

Arms

- Check lying and standing pulse (a postural increase of >30 bpm has positive LR 3.2 for large volume [>700 mL] blood loss).
- Check lying and standing BP (postural SBP drop >20 mm Hg: positive LR 1.5, negative LR 0.9; thus, not very discriminatory unless the patient is unable to stand altogether due to lightheadedness).
- Check for axillary dryness (positive LR 2.8, especially in the elderly).

HEENT

- Look for sunken eyes (positive LR 3.4), dry mucous membranes.
- Look for evidence of an elevated JVP (hypervolemia) or absent JVP when lying flat (hypovolemia).

Chest

- *Inspection*: elevated respiratory rate, use of accessory muscles indicating respiratory distress due to pulmonary edema.
- *Palpation*: displaced apex suggesting dilated cardiomyopathy.
- *Percussion*: dull percussion note suggesting a pleural effusion.
- *Auscultation*: S3 suggesting volume overload; crackles suggesting pulmonary edema.

Extremity

- Cool, pale peripheries, suggesting vasoconstriction in response to shock.
- Ankle edema, suggesting volume overload.

After the examination

- Thank the patient.
- Ensure that he is comfortable.
- Summarize your findings and offer a differential diagnosis.
- Check the patient's weight and fluid balance chart.
- Urine dipstick for increased specific gravity.
- If appropriate, indicate that you would also measure CBC, BUN, creatinine, B-type natriuretic peptide, LFTs, TFTs to help determine common etiologies of hypovolemia (blood loss vs. dehydration) or hypervolemia (heart failure, renal failure, liver failure).

Station 20

Ankle-brachial pressure index (ABPI)

Specifications: You are most likely to be requested to measure the ABPI for one arm and ankle only.

Calculating and interpreting ABPI

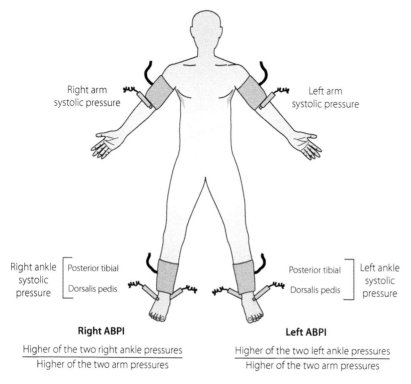

Right arm
systolic pressure

Left arm
systolic pressure

Right ankle
systolic
pressure
 — Posterior tibial
 — Dorsalis pedis

Posterior tibial
Dorsalis pedis
 — Left ankle
systolic
pressure

Right ABPI

$$\frac{\text{Higher of the two right ankle pressures}}{\text{Higher of the two arm pressures}}$$

Left ABPI

$$\frac{\text{Higher of the two left ankle pressures}}{\text{Higher of the two arm pressures}}$$

Figure 15. Calculating ABPI.

Table 6. ABPI interpretation	
ABPI	**Interpretation**
> 0.95	Normal
0.5–0.9	Claudication pain
< 0.5	Rest pain
< 0.2	Ulceration and gangrene

Cardiovascular and respiratory medicine

Before starting

- Introduce yourself to the patient.
- Explain the procedure and ask him for consent to carry it out.
- Position him at 45° with his sleeves and pants rolled up.
- Ensure that he is comfortable.
- State that you would allow him 5 minutes resting time before taking measurements.

The procedure

Brachial systolic pressure

- Place an appropriately sized cuff around the arm, as for any blood pressure recording.
- Locate the brachial pulse by palpation and apply contact gel at this site.
- Angle the hand-held Doppler probe at 45° to the skin and locate the best possible signal. Apply only gentle pressure, or else you risk occluding the artery.
- Inflate the cuff until the signal disappears.
- Progressively deflate the cuff and record the pressure at which the signal reappears.
- Repeat the procedure for the other arm or state that you would do so.
- Retain the higher of the two readings.

 Take care not to allow the probe to slide away from the line of the artery.

Ankle systolic pressure

- Place an appropriately sized cuff around the ankle immediately above the malleoli.
- Locate the dorsalis pedis pulse by palpation or with the hand-held Doppler probe and apply contact gel at this site.
- Angle the hand-held Doppler probe at 45° to the skin and locate the best possible signal. Apply only gentle pressure, or else you risk occluding the artery.
- Inflate the cuff until the signal disappears.
- Progressively deflate the cuff, and record the pressure at which the signal reappears.
- Repeat the procedure for the posterior tibial pulse, which is posterior and inferior to the medial malleolus.
- Repeat the procedure for the dorsalis pedis and posterior tibial pulses of the other ankle or state that you would do so.
- For each ankle, retain the higher of the two readings.

After the procedure

- Clean the patient's skin of contact gel and allow him time to restore his clothing.
- Clean the hand-held Doppler probe of contact gel.
- Wash your hands.
- Calculate the ABPI and explain its significance to the patient.
- Ask the patient if he has any questions or concerns.
- Thank the patient.

Station 21

Shortness of breath history

Before starting

- Introduce yourself to the patient.
- Explain that you are going to ask him some questions to uncover the nature of his shortness of breath, and ask for his consent to do this.
- Ensure that he is comfortable; if not, make sure that he is.

The history

- Name, age, and occupation.

Chief complaint

- Ask about the nature of the shortness of breath. Use open questions.
- Elicit the patient's ideas and concerns.

History of chief complaint

Ask about:

- Onset, duration, and variability of shortness of breath.
- Provoking and relieving factors.
- Severity:
  - exercise tolerance: *"How far can you walk before you get short of breath? How far could you walk before?"*
  - sleep disturbance: *"Do you get more short of breath when you lie down? How many pillows do you use?"*
  - paroxysmal nocturnal dyspnea: *"Do you wake up in the middle of the night feeling short of breath?"*
- Associated symptoms (wheeze, cough, sputum, hemoptysis, fever, night sweats, anorexia, loss of weight, lethargy, chest pain, dizziness, pedal edema).
- Effect on everyday life.
- Previous episodes of shortness of breath.
- Smoking and alcohol.

Past medical history

- Current, past, and childhood illnesses. Ask specifically about atopy (asthma/eczema/hay fever), PE/DVT, pneumonia, bronchitis, and tuberculosis.
- Previous investigations (e.g. bronchoscopy, chest X-ray).
- Surgery.

Drug history

- Prescribed medication (especially bronchodilators, NSAIDs, β-blockers, ACE inhibitors, amiodarone, and steroids).
- Over-the-counter medication.
- Recreational drugs.
- Allergies.

Cardiovascular and respiratory medicine

Family history

- Parents, siblings, and children. Focus especially on respiratory diseases such as atopy, cystic fibrosis, tuberculosis, and emphysema (α1-antitrypsin deficiency).

Social history

- Long-haul travel.
- Exposure to tuberculosis.
- Contact with asbestos.
- Contact with work-place allergens involved in, for example, baking, soldering, spray painting.
- Contact with animals, especially cats and dogs, pigeons and budgerigars.

After taking the history

- Ask the patient if there is anything else he might add that you have forgotten to ask.
- Thank the patient.
- Summarize your findings and offer a differential diagnosis.
- State that you would like to examine the patient and carry out some investigations to confirm your diagnosis.

Common conditions most likely to come up in a shortness of breath history station
Asthma: • shortness of breath, chest tightness, wheezing and coughing   • symptoms worse at night and in the early morning, and exacerbated by irritants, cold air, exercise, and emotion   • symptoms respond to bronchodilators   • there may be a history and family history of atopy
Chronic obstructive pulmonary disease: • shortness of breath, cough, wheeze   • chronic progressive disorder characterized by fixed or only partially reversible airway obstruction (cf. asthma)   • history of smoking
Pneumonia: • shortness of breath accompanied by fever, cough, and yellow sputum, and in some cases by hemoptysis and pleuritic chest pain
Tuberculosis: • shortness of breath, cough, hemoptysis, weight loss, malaise, fever, night sweats, pleural pain, symptoms of extrapulmonary disease   • more likely in certain high-risk groups such as immigrants, the homeless and the immunocompromised

Pulmonary embolism:
- shortness of breath, sometimes with pleural pain and hemoptysis
- there may be predisposing factors such as recent surgery, immobility, or long-haul travel

Lung cancer:
- symptoms may include shortness of breath, stridor, cough, hemoptysis, anorexia, weight loss, lethargy, pleural pain, hoarseness, Horner's syndrome, effects of distant metastases
- history of smoking in most cases

Heart failure:
- left ventricular failure leads to pulmonary edema
- symptoms include shortness of breath, orthopnea, paroxysmal nocturnal dyspnea, pedal edema
- there is a cough which produces pink frothy sputum

Panic attack:
- rapid onset of severe anxiety lasting for about 20–30 minutes
- associated with chest tightness and hyperventilation

Heart failure: the evidence

For heart failure	Against heart failure
• Paroxysmal nocturnal dyspnea (positive LR 2.6)	• The absence of dyspnea on exertion (negative LR 0.48)

[*JAMA* (2005), **294**: 1944–1956]

Respiratory system examination

Before starting

- Introduce yourself to the patient.
- Explain the examination and ask for his consent to carry it out.
- Position him at 45°, and ask him to remove his top(s).
- Ask him if he is in any pain or distress and ensure that he is comfortable.

The examination

General inspection

- From the end of the exam table, observe the patient's general appearance (age, state of health, nutritional status, and any other obvious signs). In particular, is he visibly short of breath or cyanosed? Does he have to sit up to breathe? Is his breathing audible? Are there any added sounds (cough, wheeze, stridor)?
- Note:
  - the rate, depth, and regularity of his breathing
  - any deformities of the chest (barrel chest, *pectus excavatum*, *pectus carinatum*) and spine
  - any asymmetry of chest expansion
  - the use of accessory muscles of respiration
  - the presence of operative scars, including in the axillae and around the back
- Next observe the surroundings. Is the patient on oxygen? If so, note the device, the concentration, and the flow rate. Look in particular for inhalers, nebulizers, peak flow meters, intravenous lines and infusions, and chest drains. If there is a sputum pot, make sure to inspect its contents.

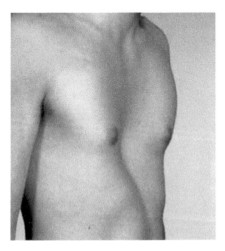

Figure 16. Respiratory system examination: *pectus excavatum.*

Inspection and examination of the hands

- Take both hands and assess them for temperature and color. Peripheral cyanosis is indicated by a bluish discoloration of the fingertips.
- Look for tar staining and finger clubbing. When the dorsum of a finger from one hand is opposed to the dorsum of a finger from the other hand, a diamond-shaped window (Schamroth's window) is formed at the base of the nailbeds. In clubbing, this diamond-shaped window is obliterated, and a distal angle is created between the fingers (see *Figure 17*). Respiratory causes of clubbing include carcinoma, fibrosing alveolitis, and chronic suppurative lung disease (see *Table 7*).
- Inspect and feel the thenar and hypothenar eminences, which can be wasted if there is an apical lung tumor that is invading or compressing the roots of the brachial plexus.
- Test for asterixis (see *Table 8*), the coarse flapping tremor of carbon dioxide retention, by asking the patient to extend both arms with the wrists in dorsiflexion and the palms facing forward. Ideally, this position should be maintained for a full 30 seconds.
- During this time, assess the radial pulse and determine its rate, rhythm, and character. Is it the bounding pulse of carbon dioxide retention?
- Indicate that you would like to measure the blood pressure.

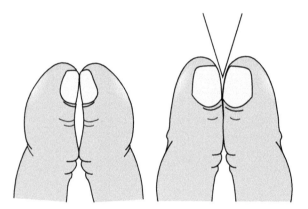

Figure 17. Clubbing. When the dorsum of a finger from one hand is opposed to the dorsum of a finger from the other hand, a diamond-shaped window is formed at the base of the nailbeds. In clubbing, this diamond-shaped window is obliterated, and a distal angle is created between the fingers.

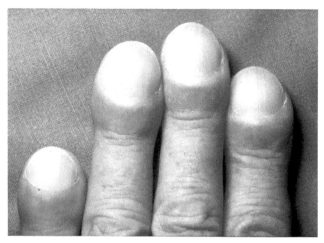

Figure 18. Finger clubbing.

Reproduced from www.mevis-research.de with permission.

Table 7. The principal causes of clubbing	
Respiratory causes	**Gastrointestinal causes**
Carcinoma	Cirrhosis
Fibrosing alveolitis	Ulcerative colitis
Chronic suppurative lung disease	Crohn's disease
Cardiac causes	Celiac disease
Infective endocarditis	**Familial**
Cyanotic heart disease	

Table 8. The principal causes of asterixis
Hepatic failure
Renal failure
Cardiac failure
Respiratory failure
Electrolyte abnormalities (hypoglycemia, hypokalemia, hypomagnesemia)
Drug intoxication, e.g. alcohol, phenytoin
CNS causes

Inspection and examination of the head and neck

- Inspect the patient's eyes. Look for a ptosis (an upper lid that encroaches upon the pupil) and for anisocoria (pupillary asymmetry). Ipsilateral ptosis, miosis, enophthalmos, and anhidrosis are strongly suggestive of Horner's syndrome, which may result from compression of the sympathetic chain by an apical lung tumor.
- Next inspect the sclera and conjunctivae for signs of anemia.
- Ask the patient to open his mouth and inspect the underside of the tongue for the blue discoloration of central cyanosis.
- Assess the jugular venous pressure (JVP) and the jugular venous pulse form (see *Station 17*). A raised JVP is suggestive of right-sided heart failure.
- Examine the lymph nodes with the patient sitting up and from behind. Have a systematic routine for examining all of the submental, submandibular, parotid, pre- and post-auricular, occipital, anterior cervical, posterior cervical, supra- and infra-clavicular, and axillary lymph nodes (see *Station 52*).
- Palpate for tracheal deviation by placing the index and middle fingers of one hand on either side of the trachea in the suprasternal notch. Alternatively, place the index and annular fingers of one hand on either clavicular head and use your middle finger (called the *Vulgaris* in Latin) to palpate the trachea.

Palpation of the chest

 Ask the patient if he has any chest pain.

- Ask the patient once again if he is in any pain. Inspect the chest more carefully, looking for asymmetries, deformities, and scars.
- Inspect the precordium and palpate for the position of the cardiac apex. Difficulty palpating for the position of the cardiac apex may indicate hyperexpansion, although this is not a specific sign.

[Note] Carry out all subsequent steps on the front of the chest and, once finished, repeat them on the back of the chest. This is far more elegant than to keep asking the patient to bend forward and backward like a Jack-in-the-box. Pulmonary anatomy is such that examination of the back of the chest yields information about the lower lobes, whereas examination of the front of the chest yields information about the upper lobes and, on the right side, also the middle lobe (*Figure 19*).

- Palpate for equal chest expansion, comparing one side to the other. Reduced unilateral chest expansion might be caused by pneumonia, pleural effusion, pneumothorax, and lung collapse. If there is a measuring tape, measure the chest expansion.

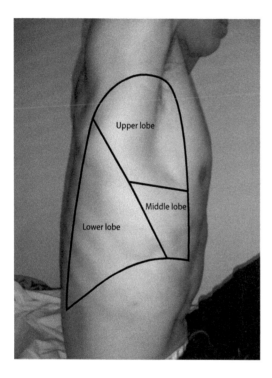

Figure 19. A right lateral view demonstrating lobar anatomy. Posterior assessment gives information about the lower lobes, whereas examination from the front looks at the upper and middle lobes (the latter only on the right).

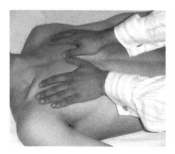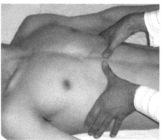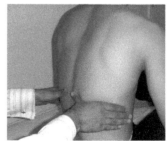

Figure 20. Palpating for equal chest expansion: upper, middle and lower lobes.

Percussion of the chest

- Percuss the chest. Start at the apex of one lung, and compare one side to the other. Do not forget to percuss over the clavicles and on the sides of the chest. For any one area, is the resonance increased or decreased? A hyper-resonant or tympanic note may indicate emphysema or pneumothorax, whereas a dull or stony dull note may indicate consolidation, fibrosis, fluid, or lung collapse. If you uncover any variation in the percussion note, be sure to map out its geographical extent.
- Test for tactile fremitus by placing the flat of the hands on the chest and asking the patient to say *"ninety nine"*.

Auscultation of the chest

- Ask the patient to take deep breaths through the mouth and, using the diaphragm of the stethoscope, auscultate the chest in the same locations as for percussion. Start at the apex of one lung, in the supraclavicular fossa, and compare one side to the other. Normal breath sounds are described as 'vesicular' and have a low pitched and rustling quality. Reduced breath sounds may indicate consolidation. Listen carefully for added sounds such as wheezes (rhonchi), crackles (crepitations), bronchial breathing, and pleural friction rubs.
- Test for vocal resonance by asking the patient to say *"ninety nine"*. Both consolidation and pleural effusions can lead to a dull percussion note, but in consolidation vocal resonance is increased whereas in pleural effusion it is decreased. Both vocal resonance and tactile fremitus (see above) provide the same sort of information.

Pneumonia: the evidence

For pneumonia
- Increased vocal resonance (Positive LR 2–8.6)

[*JAMA* (1997), **278**: 1440–1445]

Inspection and examination of the legs

- Inspect the legs for erythema and swelling. Palpate for tenderness and pitting edema. A unilateral red, swollen, and tender calf suggests a DVT, whereas bilateral swelling may indicate right-sided heart failure.

After the examination

- Look at the vital signs, examine a sputum sample, measure the peak expiratory flow rate, and order some simple investigations such as a chest X-ray and a complete blood count.
- Cover the patient up and ensure that he is comfortable.
- Thank the patient.
- Summarize your findings and offer a differential diagnosis.

Common conditions most likely to come up in a respiratory system examination station

Chronic obstructive pulmonary edema (COPD):

- signs may include shortness of breath, breathing through pursed lips, cough, hyperinflated chest, cyanosis, warm hands, tar staining, asterixis, bounding pulse, rhonchi, reduced breath sounds, signs of right heart failure (*cor pulmonale*)

Cryptogenic fibrosing alveolitis:

- signs may include shortness of breath, dry cough, cyanosis, clubbing, reduced chest expansion, fine late inspiratory crackles, signs of right heart failure (*cor pulmonale*)

Lobectomy

Abdominal pain history

Before starting

- Introduce yourself to the patient.
- Explain that you are going to ask him some questions to uncover the cause of his abdominal pain, and ask for his consent to do this.
- Ensure that he is comfortable.

 Ensure that the patient is NPO (nothing by mouth). Acute abdomen is a surgical complaint and the patient must therefore be kept NPO until the need for surgery has been excluded.

The history

- Name, age, and occupation.

Chief complaint and history of presenting illness

- For any pain, try to determine:
  - Site.
  - Onset and progression.
  - Character; for example, dull, sharp, aching, or burning.
  - Radiation.
  - Associated symptoms and signs.
  - Timing and duration.
  - Exacerbating and relieving factors.
  - Severity.
- Ensure that you ask about:
  - fever
  - loss of weight or anorexia
  - dysphagia
  - indigestion
  - nausea, vomiting, and hematemesis
  - diarrhea or constipation
  - melena or rectal bleeding
  - steatorrhea
  - jaundice
  - genitourinary symptoms: frequency, dysuria, hematuria
  - menses (menarche, menopause, length of menstrual periods, amount of bleeding, pain, intermenstrual bleeding, last menstrual period)
  - sexual activity including use of barrier methods and number of partners, to determine risk of sexually transmitted infections as a cause of abdominal pain
  - effect on everyday life

Past medical history

- Previous episodes of abdominal pain.
- Current, past, and childhood illnesses.
- Surgery.

Drug history

- Prescribed medications. Ask specifically about corticosteroids, NSAIDs, antibiotics, and the contraceptive pill.
- Over-the-counter medication.
- Recreational drugs.
- Allergies.

Family history

- Parents, siblings, and children. Ask specifically about colon cancer, irritable bowel syndrome, inflammatory bowel disease, jaundice, peptic ulcer, and polyps.

Social history

- Alcohol consumption.
- Smoking.
- Recent travel.
- Employment, past and present.
- Housing.
- Contact with jaundiced patients.

After taking the history

- Ask the patient if there is anything that he might add that you have forgotten to ask.
- Ask the patient if he has any questions or concerns.
- Thank the patient.
- In an exam, state that you would carry out a full abdominal examination and order some key investigations such as urinalysis, serum analysis, and an abdominal X-ray, as appropriate.
- Summarize your findings and offer a differential diagnosis.

Conditions most likely to come up in an abdominal pain history station
Appendicitis:
• more common in younger age groups
• diffuse central pain that then shifts into the right iliac fossa
• aggravated by movement, touch, coughing
• associated with nausea and vomiting, fever, anorexia
Gastroesophageal reflux disease:
• retrosternal burning
• clear relationship with food and alcohol, but no relationship with effort
• aggravated by lying down and alleviated by sitting up and by antacids such as Pepto-Bismol or milk
• may be associated with odynophagia and nocturnal asthma

Peptic ulceration:
- severe epigastric pain, during meals in the case of gastric ulcers, and between meals and at night in the case of duodenal ulcers
- aggravated by spicy food, alcohol, stress
- associated with bloating, heartburn, nausea and vomiting, anorexia, hematemesis, melena
- predisposed to by NSAIDs, alcohol, and smoking

Biliary colic:
- constant but episodic epigastric or right upper quadrant pain that may radiate to the back and shoulders
- can be provoked by eating a large, fatty meal
- associated with nausea and vomiting and diarrhea
- presence of fever may indicate biliary tract infection (cholecystitis)
- risk factors for gall stones are fat, forty, female, and pregnant or fertile ('the 4 Fs'), the contraceptive pill, and HRT

Acute pancreatitis:
- acute, severe epigastric pain radiating to the back
- may be alleviated by sitting forward ('pancreatic position') or by remaining still
- associated with nausea and vomiting, diarrhea, anorexia, fever

Ureteric colic:
- severe pain in the flank that radiates to the groin
- often colicky but may be constant
- associated with nausea and vomiting
- predisposed to by dehydration

Diverticulitis:
- left iliac fossa pain and tenderness
- aggravated by movement
- associated with fever, nausea, anorexia, constipation, diarrhea
- more common in the elderly

Colorectal cancer:
- signs and symptoms may include change in bowel habit, tenesmus, change in stool shape, rectal bleeding, melena, bowel obstruction leading to constipation, abdominal pain, abdominal distension, and vomiting, fatigue, anorexia, weight loss

Irritable bowel syndrome:
- chronic abdominal pain or discomfort
- associated with frequent diarrhea or constipation, bloating, urgency for bowel movements, tenesmus

 Remember that basal pneumonia, diabetic ketoacidosis, and an inferior myocardial infarct can also present as abdominal pain.

Abdominal examination

Before starting

- Introduce yourself to the patient.
- Ask the patient for permission to examine his abdomen.
- Expose the entire abdomen while paying attention to careful draping to preserve the patient's modesty.
- Position the patient so that he is lying flat on the exam table, with his arms at his side and his head supported by a pillow.
- Ensure that the patient is comfortable.

The examination

General inspection

- From the end of the exam table, observe the patient's general appearance (age, state of health, nutritional status, and any other obvious signs).
- Next observe the surroundings, looking in particular for the presence of a nasogastric tube, intravenous infusion, urinary catheter, drain, or stoma bag.
- Inspect the abdomen for its contours and any obvious distension, localized masses, scars, and skin changes. Ask the patient to lift his head up and to cough. This makes hernias more visible and, if the patient has difficulty complying with your instructions, suggests peritonism.

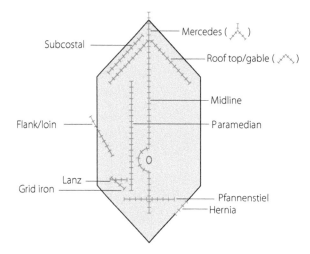

Figure 21. Abdominal scars.

Inspection and examination of the hands

- Take both hands, noting their temperature and looking for:
  - clubbing
  - palmar erythema (liver disease)
  - nail signs: leukonychia (hypoalbuminemia; see *Figure 22*) and koilonychia (iron deficiency; see *Figure 23*)
  - Dupuytren's contracture (cirrhosis; see *Figure 24*)
- Test for asterixis or 'liver flap' (hepatic failure) by showing the patient how to extend both arms with the wrists dorsiflexed and the palms facing forward. Ask him to hold this posture for at least 10 and ideally 30 seconds.

GI medicine and urology

- Next, feel the pulse for at least 15 seconds and measure the respiratory rate.
- Moving up, inspect the arms for bruising, scratch marks, injection track marks, and tattoos.

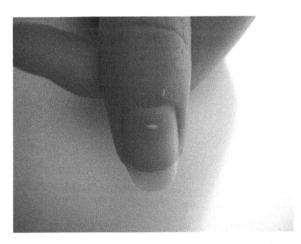

Figure 22. Leukonychia.
Reproduced from http://commons.wikimedia.org with permission.

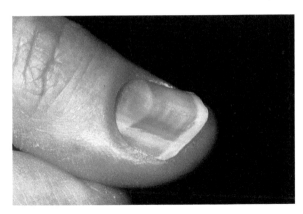

Figure 23. Koilonychia.
Photograph by Dr P. Marazzi, reproduced with permission from Science Photo Library.

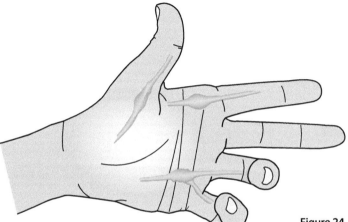

Figure 24. Dupuytren's contracture.

Inspection and examination of the head, neck, and upper body

- Ask the patient to look up and then inspect the sclera for jaundice.
- Gently retract the eyelid and inspect the conjunctiva for anemia.
- Ask the patient to open his mouth, and note any odor on the breath (alcohol, *fetor hepaticus*, ketones). Inspect the mouth, looking for signs of dehydration, furring of the tongue (loss of appetite), angular stomatitis (nutritional deficiency), atrophic glossitis (iron deficiency, vitamin B12 deficiency, folate deficiency; see *Figure 25*), ulcers (Crohn's disease), and the state of the dentition.
- If you suspect alcoholism or an eating disorder, feel for enlargement of the parotid glands.
- Assess the jugular venous pressure (JVP).
- Palpate the neck for lymphadenopathy, making sure to evaluate the left supraclavicular fossa (Virchow's node, also known as Troisier's sign, gastric carcinoma).
- Examine the upper body for gynecomastia (cirrhosis), caput medusae, and spider nevi (chronic liver disease).

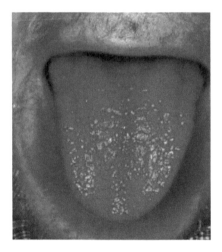

Figure 25. Atrophic glossitis. Note the loss of filliform papillae.
Reproduced from www.joplink.net – photograph by Dr Echenique-Eligondo.

Palpation of the abdomen

 Before you begin, ask the patient to identify any area of pain or tenderness.

- Sit or kneel beside the patient and use the palmar surface of your fingers to lightly palpate in all nine regions of the abdomen (*Figure 26*), beginning with the region furthest away from any pain or tenderness. By flexing and extending your metacarpophalangeal joints, palpate for tenderness, rebound tenderness, guarding, and rigidity. Keep looking at the patient's face for any signs of discomfort.
- Repeat the procedure, this time palpating more deeply so as to localize and describe any masses.

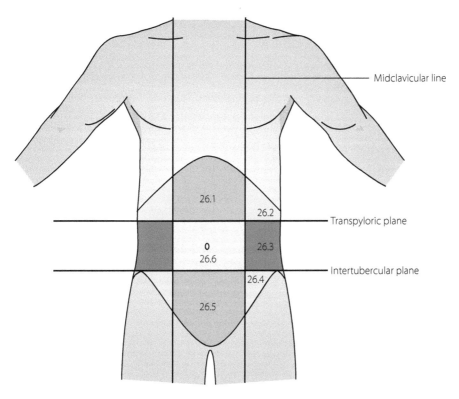

Figure 26. Regions of the abdomen.
  26.1 Epigastric
  26.2 Left hypochondriac
  26.3 Left lumbar
  26.4 Left iliac fossa
  26.5 Suprapubic/hypogastric
  26.6 Umbilical

In the figure: Midclavicular line, Transpyloric plane, Intertubercular plane

Palpation of the organs

- *Liver* – Ask the patient to breathe in and out and, starting in the right iliac fossa, feel for the inferior liver edge using the radial aspect of your index finger. Each time the patient inspires, move your hand closer to the costal margin and press your fingers firmly into the abdominal wall. The inferior liver edge may be felt as the liver descends upon inspiration, and can be described in terms of regularity, nodularity, and tenderness.
- *Gallbladder* – Palpate for tenderness over the tip of the right ninth rib.
- *Spleen* – Palpate for the spleen as for the liver, once again starting in the right iliac fossa. Press the tips of your fingers firmly against the abdominal wall so that your hand is pointing up and leftward. If the spleen is enlarged, the splenic notch may be 'caught' as the spleen descends upon inspiration.
- *Kidneys* – Position the patient close to the edge of the bed and ballot each kidney using the technique of deep bimanual palpation. Place one hand flat over the anterior aspect of the flank (right hand for left kidney, left hand for right kidney), and press down while using the other hand to push the kidney up from below.
- *Aorta* – Palpate the descending aorta with the tips of your fingers on either side of the midline, just above the umbilicus. Pressing your fingers firmly into the abdominal wall, assess whether

the aorta is pulsatile and whether it is expansile, i.e. whether it causes the fingers of your right and left hands to move apart.

Abdominal aortic aneurysm (AAA): the evidence
• It is the width of the palpable aorta that determines whether an AAA is present.
• A palpable aorta > 2.5 cm increases the likelihood of an AAA.
For an AAA
• Palpable aortic diameter ≥ 3 cm (Positive LR 12)
[*JAMA* (1999), **281**: 77–82]

Percussion

- *Liver* – Percuss out the entire craniocaudal extent of the liver. In the mid-clavicular line, start above the right fifth intercostal space and progress downward. The normal liver represents an area of dullness which typically extends from the fifth intercostal space to the edge of the costal margin. Beyond this point, the abdomen should be resonant to percussion.
- *Spleen* – As for the liver, percuss the spleen to determine its size.
- *Bladder* – Percuss the suprapubic area for the undue dullness of bladder distension.
- *'Shifting dullness'* – this sign indicates ascites. Percuss down the right side of the abdomen. If an area of dullness is detected, keep two fingers on it and ask the patient to roll over onto his left. After about 30 seconds, re-percuss the area which should now sound resonant. The change in the percussion note reflects the redistribution of ascitic fluid under the effect of gravity.
- *'Fluid thrill'* – this sign indicates severe ascites. Ask the patient to place his hand along the midline of his abdomen. Then place one hand on one flank, and flick the opposite flank with your other hand in an attempt to elicit a thrill.

Auscultation

Auscultate over:

- The mid-abdomen for bowel sounds (*Table 9*). Listen for 30 seconds before concluding that they are normal, hyperactive, hypoactive, or absent.
- The abdominal aorta for aortic bruits suggestive of arteriosclerosis or an aneurysm.
- 2.5 cm above and lateral to the umbilicus for renal artery bruits suggestive of renal artery stenosis.

Table 9. Principal causes of altered bowel sounds	
Hypoactive	• Constipation
	• Drugs such as anticholinergics and opiates
	• General anesthesia
	• Abdominal surgery
	• Paralytic ileus (absent bowel sounds)
Hyperactive	• Diarrhea of any cause
	• Inflammatory bowel disease
	• GI bleeding
	• Mechanical bowel obstruction (high pitched bowel sounds)

After the examination

- Cover up the patient and thank him. Enquire about and address any concerns that he may have.
- In an exam, indicate to the examiner that you would normally test for pedal edema, examine the hernia orifices and the external genitalia, and carry out a digital rectal examination. You would also look at the vital signs, dipstick the urine, and consider investigations such as ultrasound scan, CBC, LFTs, BUN and electrolytes, clotting screen, pregnancy test, and urine drug screen.
- Summarize your findings and offer a differential diagnosis.

Conditions most likely to come up in an abdominal examination station
Chronic liver disease: • may result from alcoholic liver disease, viral hepatitis, right heart failure, hemochromatosis, Wilson's disease, amongst others   • signs may include clubbing, palmar erythema, leukonychia, metabolic flap, hyperventilation, bruising, jaundice, gynecomastia, spider nevi, caput medusae, scratch marks, hepatomegaly, ascites, pedal edema, Dupuytren's contracture (alcohol), tattoos (hepatitis C), signs of right heart failure such as raised JVP and pedal edema, bronzing of the skin (hemochromatosis), Kayser–Fleischer rings (Wilson's disease)
Splenomegaly: • causes include portal hypertension (usually complicating liver cirrhosis), lymphoproliferative and myeloproliferative diseases, hemolytic anemias, and infections such as infectious mononucleosis and malaria
Polycystic kidney
Renal transplant
Scars
Hernias (see *Station 26*)

Station 25

Rectal examination

Rectal examination is commonly indicated in cases of rectal or GI bleeding (suspected or actual), severe constipation, fecal or urinary incontinence, anal or rectal pain, suspected enlargement of the prostate gland, and urethral discharge or bleeding. It can also be used to screen for cancers of the rectum, colon, and prostate.

Specifications: A plastic model in lieu of a patient.

Before starting

- Introduce yourself to the patient.
- Explain the procedure to him, emphasizing that it might be uncomfortable but that it should not be painful, and ask for his consent to carry it out.
- Ask for a chaperone.
- Ensure privacy.
- Ask the patient to lower his pants and underpants.
- Ask him to lie on his left side, to bring his buttocks to the side of the exam table, and to bring his knees up to his chest.

The examination

- Put on a pair of gloves.
- Gently separate the buttocks and inspect the anus and surrounding skin. In particular, note any skin tags, excoriations, ulcers, fissures, external hemorrhoids, prolapsed hemorrhoids, and mucosal prolapse.
- Lubricate the index finger of your right hand using sterile water-soluble lubricant.
- Position the finger over the anus, as if pointing to the genitalia.
- Ask the patient to bear down so as to relax the anal sphincter.
- Gently insert the finger into the anus, through the anal canal, and into the rectum (*Figure 27*). Note any pain upon insertion.

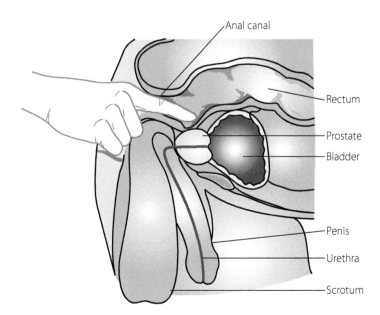

Anal canal

Rectum

Prostate

Bladder

Penis

Urethra

Scrotum

Figure 27. Digital rectal examination.

- Test anal tone by asking the patient to squeeze your finger.
- Rotate the finger so as to palpate the entire circumference of the anal canal and rectum. Feel for any masses, ulcers, or induration and for feces in the rectum. If there are any feces in the rectum, assess their consistency.
  - In males pay specific attention to the size, shape, surface, and consistency of the prostate gland. Assess whether the midline groove is palpable.
  - In females, the cervix and uterus may be palpable.
- Remove the finger and examine the glove. In particular look at the color of any stool, and for the presence of any mucus or blood.
- Remove and dispose of the gloves.

After the examination

- Clean off any lubricant or feces on the anus or anal margin.
- Give the patient time to put his clothes back on.
- Ensure that he is comfortable.
- Address any questions or concerns that he may have.
- In an exam, present your findings to the examiner, and offer a differential diagnosis.

Conditions most likely to come up in a rectal examination station
Benign prostatic hypertrophy (BPH):
• in BPH the prostate is enlarged in size (>3.5 cm) and slightly distorted in shape, but it is still rubbery and firm, with a smooth surface and a palpable midline groove
Prostate carcinoma
• in prostate carcinoma, the prostate is also enlarged and asymmetrical, but this time it is hard and irregular/nodular and the midline groove may no longer be palpable

Hernia examination

Inguinal anatomy

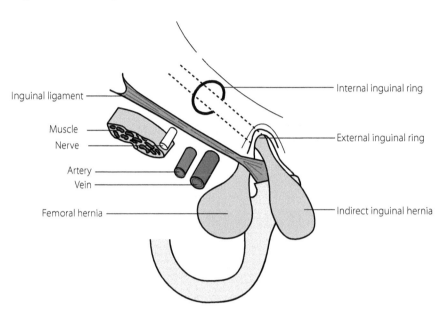

Figure 28. The inguinal canal runs along the inguinal ligament, from the internal (deep) ring to the external (superficial) ring. The inguinal ligament stretches from the anterior superior iliac spine to the pubic tubercle. The internal ring lies approximately 1.5 cm superior to the femoral pulse, itself in the midline of the inguinal ligament. The external ring lies immediately superior and medial to the pubic tubercle.

Definition of a hernia

A hernia is defined as the protrusion of an organ or part thereof through a deficiency in the wall of the cavity in which it is contained. There are many different types of hernia but the ones that are most likely to be encountered in clinical practice or to be examined and discussed in an exam are indirect and direct inguinal hernias and femoral hernias. Their principal differentiating features are summarized in *Table 10*. The differential diagnosis of a lump in the groin is listed in *Table 11*.

Table 10. Principal differentiating features of indirect and direct inguinal and femoral hernias		
Indirect hernia	**Direct hernia**	**Femoral hernia**
• Neck of hernia is superior to the inguinal ligament/pubic tubercle and lateral to the inferior epigastric vessels • Accounts for 80% of inguinal hernias • Irreducible • Can strangulate	• Neck of hernia is superior to the inguinal ligament/ pubic tubercle and medial to the inferior epigastric vessels • Accounts for 20% of inguinal hernias • Easily reducible • Rarely strangulates	• Neck of hernia is inferior and lateral to the inguinal ligament pubic tubercle • Is more common in females • Often irreducible • Frequently strangulates

Table 11. Differential diagnosis of a lump in the groin	
Superior to the inguinal ligament	**Inferior to the inguinal ligament**
• Indirect or direct inguinal hernia • Incisional hernia • Sebaceous cyst • Lipoma • Undescended testis	• Femoral hernia • Lymph node • Sebaceous cyst • Lipoma • Saphena varix • Femoral artery aneurysm • Psoas abscess (rare) • Undescended testis • Scrotal mass (see *Station 28*)

Before starting

- Introduce yourself to the patient.
- Explain the examination and ask for his consent to carry it out.
- Ask for a chaperone.
- Ask the patient to lie on the exam table and to expose his abdomen from the umbilicus to the knees.
- Ensure that he is comfortable.
- Warm up your hands.

 Ensure the patient's dignity at all times.

The examination

Inspection and palpation

- Inspect the groins (both sides!) for an obvious lump. If a lump is visible, determine its location in relation to its surrounding anatomical landmarks. Also determine its size, shape, color, consistency, and mobility. Is it tender to touch? Can it be transilluminated? (See *Station 52: Examination of a superficial mass*.)
- Look for old surgical scars (incisional hernia).
- Ask the patient to stand up and look again.

Cough impulse and cough tests

(The patient is still standing.)

- Ask the patient to cough and look again.
- Test the lump for a cough impulse. Place two fingers over the lump and ask the patient to cough once more.
- If you are satisfied that the lump is an inguinal hernia, ask the patient to reduce the lump. Once the lump is fully reduced, place two fingers over the internal ring and ask the patient to cough.
  - If the lump does not reappear it is an indirect inguinal hernia. Release your fingers and ask the patient to cough again.
  - If the lump reappears medially it is a direct inguinal hernia.
- Once again ask the patient to reduce the lump. This time place two fingers over the *external* ring and ask the patient to cough.

- – If the lump does not reappear it is a direct inguinal hernia. Release your fingers and ask the patient to cough again.
  - – If the lump reappears laterally it is an indirect inguinal hernia.
- Percuss the lump for resonance (bowel involvement).
- Auscultate the lump for bowel sounds (bowel involvement).

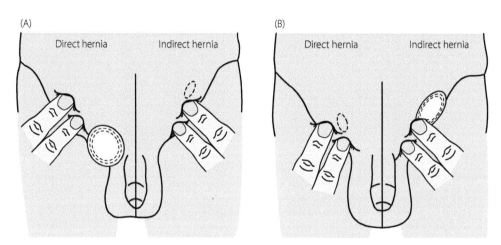

Figure 29. The cough test with two fingers over the internal ring (A) and then over the external ring (B).

After the examination

- Indicate that you would also examine the femoral pulses, inguinal lymph nodes, and scrotum.
- Cover up the patient.
- Ensure that he is comfortable.
- Thank him.
- In an exam summarize your findings and offer a differential diagnosis. Don't fret over your diagnosis as even experienced surgeons are notoriously poor at differentiating between indirect and direct inguinal hernias. Apart from inguinal and femoral hernias, other (more rare) types of hernia are epigastric hernias that occur in the epigastric area in the midline, spigellian or semilunar hernias that occur on the outer border of the rectus muscles, umbilical and para-umbilical hernias that occur at or around the navel, and incisional hernias that occur at the site of an old surgical incision.
- Wash your hands.

Urological history

Before starting

- Introduce yourself to the patient.
- Explain that you are going to ask him some questions to uncover the nature of his urological complaint, and ask for consent to do this.
- Ensure that he is comfortable.

The history

- Name, age, and occupation.

Chief complaint and history of presenting illness

- Ask about the chief complaint. Ask open questions.
- Elicit the patient's ideas, concerns, and expectations.
- Determine the time course of events and the severity of the problem.
- Ask specifically about:
  - pain: for any pain, ask about site, radiation, intensity, character, onset, duration, relieving and aggravating factors, and associated factors
  - fever
  - frequency: *"Are you urinating more often than usual?"*
  - nocturia: *"Do you find yourself waking up in the middle of the night to urinate?"*
  - urgency: *"When you need to urinate, how long can you wait?"*
  - incontinence: *"Are there times when it can no longer wait and you end up going there and then?"*
  - dysuria: *"When you urinate, is there any pain or burning?"*
  - hematuria: *"When you urinate, is there any blood in your urine? Does it color all of your urine or only some of it?"*
  - hesitancy, poor stream and terminal dribbling (if male): *"When you are standing at the toilet do you have to wait before you are able to urinate? Is the jet as strong as it ever was? What about after, does urine continue to trickle out?"*
  - back pain, leg weakness, weight loss, nausea, anorexia
  - vaginal/urethral discharge, genital sores
  - testicular masses, testicular pain
  - sexual dysfunction
  - sexual contacts

Past medical history

- Past urological problems.
- Ask specifically about UTI, renal colic, diabetes mellitus, hypertension, and gout.
- Current, past, and childhood illnesses.
- Surgery.

Drug history

- Prescribed medication including anticholinergics and anticoagulants.
- Over-the-counter medication.
- Recreational drugs.
- Allergies.

Family history

- Parents, siblings, and children. In particular, has anyone in the family had a similar problem?
- Ask specifically about polycystic kidney disease and bladder cancer.

Social history

- Employment. Has the patient ever worked with chemicals or dyes?
- Housing.
- Travel.
- Alcohol consumption.
- Smoking.

After taking the history

- Ask the patient if there is anything he might add that you have forgotten to ask about.
- Thank the patient.
- In an exam, state that you would carry out abdominal and genital examinations and order some key investigations, e.g. urine dipstick, urine microscopy and culture, BUN and electrolytes, transrectal ultrasound, cystoscopy, KUB X-ray as indicated.
- Summarize your findings and offer a differential diagnosis.

UTI in women: the evidence

For UTI in women	Against UTI in women
• Dysuria and frequency without vaginal discharge or irritation (positive LR 24.6).	• Vaginal discharge (negative LR 0.3) or vaginal irritation (negative LR 0.2).

[*JAMA* (2002), **287**: 2701–2710]

Conditions most likely to come up in a urological history station

Urinary tract infection:

- most common in young females
- common symptoms are frequency, urgency, dysuria, hematuria, and a pressure above the pubic bone
- if the infection is above the bladder, there may be fever, nausea, and back pain
- there may be history of recent sexual intercourse

Benign prostatic hypertrophy:

- most common in elderly males
- common symptoms are frequency, nocturia, urgency, incontinence, hesitancy, poor stream and intermittency, and terminal dribbling

Prostate carcinoma:

- most common in elderly males
- symptoms, when present, are similar to those seen in benign prostatic hypertrophy with the possible addition of dysuria, hematuria, sexual dysfunction, weight loss, and bone pain
- there may be a family history

Bladder carcinoma:

- three to four times more common in males than in females
- more common in the elderly
- painless hematuria is characteristic, but there may also be dysuria and/or frequency
- associated with smoking and occupational exposure to chemicals and dyes

Renal calculus:

- more common in males than in females
- severe pain in the flank that radiates to the groin
- the pain is often colicky but it may be constant
- the pain may be associated with nausea and vomiting
- hematuria is a common finding
- dehydration is a common predisposing factor

Male genitalia examination

Specifications: In an exam, you may be asked to examine the male genitalia on a real patient or, more likely, on a pelvic mannequin.

Before starting

- Introduce yourself to the patient.
- Explain the examination and ask for his consent to carry it out.
- Ask for a chaperone.
- Ask him to lie on the exam table and expose his groin area.
- Ensure that he is comfortable.

 Ensure the patient's comfort and dignity at all times.

The examination

General inspection

- From the end of the exam table observe the patient's general appearance. The patient's age can give you an indication of the most likely pathology.
- In particular, note the distribution of facial, axillary, and pubic hair.
- Look for gynecomastia.

Inspection and examination of the male genitalia

- Warm your hands.
- Ensure that the patient is not in pain.

Penis

- Inspect the penis for lesions and ulcers.
- Retract the foreskin, if present, and examine the *glans penis* and the external urethral meatus. Is there a discharge? Can a discharge be expressed?
  - If there is a discharge, indicate that you would swab it for microscopy and culture.

Scrotum

- Inspect the scrotum. Are the testicles present? Is their lie normal? If a testicle is absent, is it retracted or undescended? If you find a scar, the absent testicle may have been surgically removed.
- Fix upon the patient's face and palpate:
  - the testis
  - the epididymis
  - the spermatic cord
- If you locate a mass, try to get above it. If you cannot, it is likely to be a hernia so test for a cough impulse (see *Station 26*). Determine the size, shape and consistency of the mass.
- Next, transilluminate the mass using a pen flashlight. Is it a cyst or a solid mass? If it is a cyst, is it a hydrocele or an epididymal cyst? If it is a solid mass, is it tender? Is it testicular or epididymal?
- If you suspect a varicocele, a collection of varicosities in the pampiniform venous plexus, examine the patient in the standing position and test for a cough impulse. **Note that varicoceles are almost invariably left-sided.**

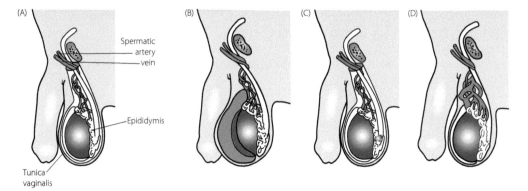

Figure 30. Normal testis and appendages (A), hydrocele (B), epididymal cyst (C), and varicocele (D).

Examination of the lymphatics

- Palpate the inguinal nodes in the inguinal crease. Remember that only the penis and scrotum drain to the inguinal nodes, as the testicles drain to the para-aortic lymph nodes.

After the examination

- Cover up the patient.
- Thank the patient.
- Ensure that he is comfortable.
- Summarize your findings and offer a differential diagnosis.

Conditions most likely to come up in a male genitalia examination	
Hydrocele: - collection of fluid in the tunica vaginalis surrounding the testis - presents as unilateral (or less commonly bilateral) scrotal swelling - not tender - fluctuant - transilluminant	**Varicocele:** - dilated veins along the spermatic cord - almost invariably left-sided - 'bag of worms' upon palpation - there may be a cough impulse - likely to disappear upon lying down
Epididymal cyst: - arises in the epididymis - epididymal cysts may be multiple and bilateral - unlike in a hydrocele, the testis is palpable quite separately from the cyst - smooth and fluctuant - transilluminant	**Direct inguinal hernia** (see *Station 26*)

History of headaches

'I'm very brave generally', he went on in a low voice: 'only today I happen to have a headache'.

Lewis Carroll, *Through the Looking Glass*

Before starting

- Introduce yourself to the patient.
- Explain that you are going to ask him some questions to uncover the nature of his headaches, and ask for his consent to do this.
- Ensure that he is comfortable.

The history

- Name, age, and occupation.

Chief complaint and history of presenting illness

First use open questions to get the patient's history, and elicit his ideas, concerns, and expectations.

Then ask specifically about:

- **S**ite. Ask the patient to point at the site of the pain.
- **O**nset.
- **C**haracter, for example, sharp, dull, throbbing, band-like constriction.
- **R**adiation.
- **A**ssociated factors.
  - Nausea and vomiting.
  - Visual disturbances such as double vision and fortification spectra.
  - Photophobia.
  - Fever, chills.
  - Weight loss.
  - Rash.
  - Scalp tenderness.
  - Neck pain, stiffness.
  - Myalgia.
  - Rhinorrhea, lacrimation.
  - Altered mental status.
  - Neurological deficit (weakness, numbness, 'pins and needles').
- **T**iming and duration.
- **E**xacerbating and relieving factors, for example, activity, stress, eye strain, caffeine, alcohol, dehydration, hunger, certain foods, coughing/sneezing).
- **S**everity. Ask the patient to rate the pain on a scale of 1 to 10, and to determine the effect that it is having on his life.

Past medical history

- Current, past, and childhood illnesses.
- Ask specifically about headache, migraine, hypertension, cardiovascular disease, and travel sickness as a child.
- Surgery.

Drug history

- Prescribed medication. Ask specifically about withdrawal from NSAIDs, opioids, nitroglycerin, and calcium channel blockers.
- Over-the-counter medication.
- Recreational drugs.
- Allergies.

Family history

- Parents, siblings, and children.
- Ask about migraine and travel sickness.

Social history

- Employment, past and present.
- Housing.
- Mood. Depression is a common cause of headaches.
- Smoking.
- Alcohol use. Alcohol is a common cause of headaches.
- Diet: tea and coffee, cheese and yogurt, chocolate.

After taking the history

- Ask the patient if there is anything he might like to add that you have forgotten to ask about.
- Ask him if he has any questions or concerns.
- Thank him.
- Summarize your findings and offer a differential diagnosis.
- In an exam, state that you would like to carry out a physical examination and some investigations to confirm your diagnosis and exclude life-threatening causes of headaches (see box below).

Neurology

Conditions most likely to come up in a history of headaches station

Tension headaches:
- constant pressure, 'as if the head were being squeezed in a vise'
- pain typically last 4–6 hours but this is highly variable
- may be precipitated by stress, eye strain, sleep deprivation, bad posture, irregular meal times

Cluster headaches ('suicide headaches'):
- excruciating unilateral headache that is of rapid onset
- located in the periorbital or temple area, may radiate to the neck or shoulder
- associated with autonomic symptoms such as ptosis, conjunctival injection, lacrimation
- each headache lasts from 15 minutes to 3 hours
- headaches most often occur in 'clusters': once or more every day, often at the same time of day, for a period of several weeks

Migraines:
- unilateral, dull, throbbing headache lasting from 4 to 72 hours
- may be aggravated by activity
- associated with nausea, vomiting, photophobia, phonophobia
- about half experience prodromal symptoms such as altered mood, irritability, or fatigue several hours or days before the headache
- about one-third experience an aura, commonly consisting of visual disturbances or neurological symptoms, before or along with the headache
- frequency of headaches varies considerably, but average is about 1–3 a month

Cranial arteritis:
- unilateral pain in the temporal region
- associated with scalp tenderness, jaw claudication, blurred vision, and tinnitus
- three times more common in females
- mean age of onset is 70 years
- urgent treatment is required to prevent sudden loss of vision

Cervical spondylosis:
- occipital headaches associated with cervical pain
- cervical pain may radiate to the base of the skull, shoulder, or hand and fingers
- may be associated with weakness, numbness, or pins and needles in the arms and hands

Meningitis:
- severe and bilateral headache
- may be associated with high fever, neck stiffness, photophobia, phonophobia, altered mental status

Subarachnoid hemorrhage:
- thunderclap headache ('like being kicked in the head') that is of very rapid onset
- may be associated with vomiting, altered mental status, neck stiffness, photophobia, visual disturbances, seizures

Raised intracranial pressure
- dull, throbbing headache associated with vomiting, ocular palsies, visual disturbances, altered mental status
- may be worse in the morning and may wake the patient up from sleep
- aggravated by coughing and head movement
- alleviated by standing

Sinusitis:
- dull and constant headache or facial pain over the sinuses
- may be associated with flu-like symptoms and facial tenderness
- may be aggravated by bending over or lying down

Trigeminal neuralgia:
- intense unilateral facial pain ('like stabbing electric shocks') lasting from seconds to minutes
- may occur several times a day
- triggered by common activities such as eating, talking, shaving, and tooth-brushing
- may be associated with a trigger area on the face

Migraine: the evidence

For migraine

- If 4/5 of **P**ounding, duration 4–72 h**O**urs, **U**nilateral, **N**ausea, **D**isabling (POUNDing) positive LR 24; if 3/5 positive LR 3.5

[*JAMA* (2006), **296**: 1274–1283]

Station 30

History of collapse

Before starting

- Introduce yourself to the patient.
- Explain that you are going to ask him some questions to uncover the cause of his collapse, and ask for his consent to do this.
- Ensure that he is comfortable.

The history

- Name, age, and occupation.

Chief complaint and history of presenting illness

First use open questions to get the patient's story, and elicit their ideas, concerns and expectations.

Think about the common causes of a collapse, as these should inform your line of questioning.

Ask about:

- If the patient remembers falling.
- The circumstances of the fall:
  - had the patient just arisen from bed? (postural hypotension)
  - did the patient suffer an intense emotion? (vasovagal syncope)
  - had the patient been coughing or straining? (situational syncope)
  - had the patient been turning or extending his neck? (carotid sinus syncope)
  - had the patient been exercising? (arrhythmia)
  - did the patient have any palpitations, chest pain, or shortness of breath? (arrhythmia)
- Any loss of consciousness and its duration.
- Prodromal symptoms such as aura, change in mood, strange feeling in the gut, sensation of *déjà vu*.
- Fitting, frothing at the mouth, tongue biting, incontinence.
- Headache or confusion, or amnesia upon recovery.
- Injuries sustained.
- Previous episodes.

Past medical history

- Current, past, and childhood illnesses. Ask specifically about epilepsy, hypertension, heart problems, stroke, diabetes (autonomic neuropathy), cervical spondylosis, and arthritis.
- Surgery.

Drug history

- Prescribed medication. Drugs such as antipsychotics, tricyclic antidepressants, and antihypertensives can cause postural hypotension. Insulin can cause hypoglycemia.
- Over-the-counter medication.
- Recreational drugs.
- Recent changes in medication.

Family history

- Parents, siblings, and children.
- Ask specifically about epilepsy and heart problems.

Social history

- Smoking.
- Alcohol use.
- Employment, past and present.
- Housing.
- Effect of falls on patient's life.

After taking the history

- Ask the patient if there is anything he might add that you have forgotten to ask about.
- Ask him if he has any questions or concerns.
- Thank him.
- Summarize your findings and offer a differential diagnosis.
- In an exam, state that you would like to carry out a physical examination and some investigations to confirm your diagnosis.

Conditions most likely to appear in a history of collapse station	
Simple faint:	**Postural hypotension:**
• loss of consciousness lasting from a few seconds to a few minutes is preceded by nausea, sweatiness, dizziness or tightness in the throat • provoked by stressful, anxiety-provoking, or painful situations (vasovagal syncope), by coughing or straining (situational syncope), or by applying pressure upon the carotid sinus, for example, by wearing a tight collar, turning the head, or shaving (carotid sinus syncope)	• loss of consciousness preceded by dizziness, light-headedness, confusion, or blurry vision • provoked by postural change • causes include hypovolemia (e.g. dehydration, bleeding, diuretics, vasodilators), drugs (e.g. tricyclic antidepressants, antipsychotics, alpha blockers), and certain medical conditions (e.g. diabetes, Addison's disease)

Arrhythmia (cardiac syncope):

- may be either a bradycardia or tachycardia
- may be provoked by exertion
- may be associated with palpitations, chest pain, shortness of breath, fatigue
- history of heart disease/risk factors for heart disease are very likely
- patient should be hospitalized and placed on a cardiac monitor to rule out ventricular tachycardia, which can result in sudden death
- less commonly, cardiac syncope can be caused by an obstructive cardiac lesion such as aortic or mitral stenosis

Generalized tonic-clonic seizure:

- sudden loss of consciousness accompanied by fitting, frothing at the mouth, tongue biting, incontinence
- seizure lasts for about 2 minutes
- seizure is followed by confusion and amnesia
- seizure may be preceded by an aura which may involve déjà vu, dizziness, unusual emotions, altered sense perceptions, or other symptoms

Transient ischemic attack:

- most frequent symptoms include loss of vision, aphasia, unilateral hemiparesis, and unilateral paresthesia
- symptoms last for a few seconds to a few minutes and never for more than 24 hours (by definition)
- loss of consciousness can occur, although it is very uncommon

Cranial nerve examination

Specifications: In an exam, you may be asked to limit your examination to certain cranial nerves only, e.g. I–VI, VII–XII.

Before starting

- Introduce yourself to the patient.
- Explain the examination and ask for his consent to carry it out.
- Ensure that he is comfortable.

The examination

The olfactory nerve (CN I)

- Ask the patient if he has noticed a change in his sense of smell or taste. If he has, indicate that you would perform an olfactory examination by asking the patient to smell different scents, such as mint or coffee.

Junior Resident's tips
To remember the steps of CN II exam: **A**cuity **F**ields **R**eflexes **O**phthalmoscopy (**AFRO**)

The optic nerve (CN II)

(See *Station 46: Vision and the eye examination* for more details.)

- Ask the patient whether he wears glasses. If he does, ask him to put them on.
- Test visual acuity on a Snellen chart either from a distance of 6 or 3 meters.
- Test near vision by asking the patient to read test types (or a page in a book).
- Indicate that you could use Ishihara plates to test color vision specifically.
- Test the visual fields by confrontation. Sit directly opposite the patient, at the same level as him. Ask him to look straight at you and to cover his right eye with his right hand. Cover your left eye with your left hand, and test the visual field of his left eye with your right hand. Bring a wiggly finger into the upper left quadrant, asking the patient to say when he sees the finger. Repeat for the lower left quadrant. Then swap hands and test the upper and lower right quadrants. Now ask the patient to cover his left eye with his left hand. Cover your right eye with your right hand and test the visual field of his right eye with your left hand. Bring a wiggly finger into the upper right quadrant, asking the patient to say when he sees the finger. Repeat for the lower right quadrant. Then swap hands and test the upper and lower left quadrants.
- Indicate that you could use a red hat pin to uncover the blind spot and the presence of a central scotoma.
- Indicate that you could examine the eyes by direct fundoscopy.

Neurology

Clinical Skills for Medical Students

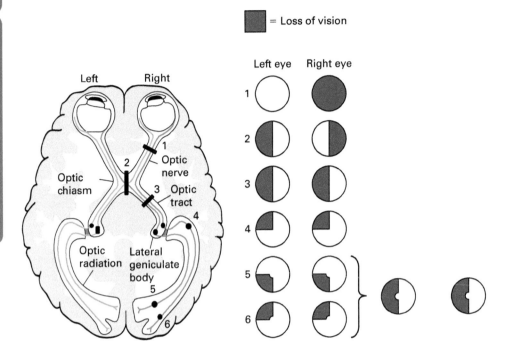

Figure 31. Visual field defects and their origins.

The oculomotor, trochlear, and abducens nerves (CN III, IV, and VI)

(See *Station 46: Vision and the eye examination* for more details.)

- Inspect the eyes, paying particular attention to the size and symmetry of the pupils, and excluding a visible ptosis (Horner's syndrome; see *Figure 32*) or squint.
- Test the direct and consensual pupillary light reflexes. Explain that you are going to shine a bright light into the patient's eye and that this may feel uncomfortable. Bring the light in onto his left eye and look for pupil constriction. Bring the light in onto his left eye once again, but this time look for pupil constriction in his *right eye* (consensual reflex). Repeat for the right eye.
- Perform the swinging flashlight test. Swing the light from one eye to another and look for sustained pupil constriction in both eyes. Intermittent pupil constriction in one eye (Marcus Gunn pupil) suggests a lesion of the optic nerve anterior to the optic chiasm.
- Perform the cover test. Ask the patient to fixate on a point and cover one eye. Observe the movement of the uncovered eye. Repeat the test for the other eye.
- Examine eye movements. Ask the patient to keep his head still and to follow your finger with his eyes. Ask him to report any pain or double vision at any point. Draw an 'H' shape with your finger. Observe for nystagmus at the extremes of gaze.
- Test the accommodation reflex. Ask the patient to follow your finger in to his nose. As the eyes converge, the pupils should constrict.

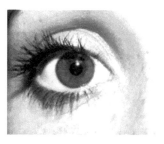
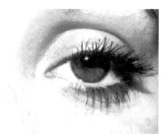

Figure 32. Horner's syndrome. Characteristic features are ipsilateral ptosis, miosis, apparent enophthalmos, and anhidrosis and vasodilatation on the same side of the face.

Reproduced from Otolaryngology – Houston at www.ghorayeb.com with permission.

Neurology

The trigeminal nerve (CN V)

Sensory part

- Using cotton wool, test light touch in the three branches of the trigeminal nerve. Compare both sides.
- Indicate that you could test the corneal reflex, but that this is likely to cause the patient some discomfort.

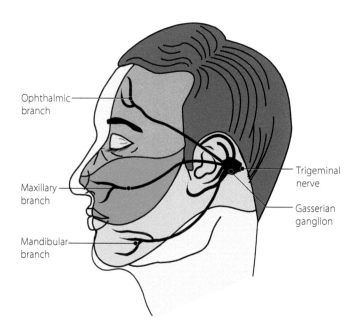

Figure 33. The three branches of the trigeminal nerve. 'Trigeminal' means 'three twins'.

Motor part

- Test the muscles of mastication (the temporalis, masseter, and pterygoid muscles) by asking the patient to:
  - clench his teeth (palpate his temporalis and masseter muscles bilaterally)
  - open and close his mouth against resistance (place your fist under his chin)
- Indicate that you could test the jaw jerk. Ask the patient to let his mouth fall open slightly. Place your fingers on the top of his mandible and tap them lightly with a reflex hammer.

The facial nerve (CN VII)

- Look for facial asymmetry. Note that the nasolabial folds and the angle of the mouth are especially indicative of facial asymmetry.

Sensory part

- Indicate that you could test the anterior two-thirds of the tongue for taste.

Motor part

- Test the muscles of facial expression by asking the patient to:
  - lift his eyebrows as far as they will go
  - close his eyes as tightly as possible (try to open them)
  - blow out his cheeks
  - purse his lips or whistle
  - show his teeth

The acoustic nerve (CN VIII)

(See *Station 45: Hearing and the ear examination* for more details.)

- Test hearing sensitivity in each ear by occluding one ear and rubbing your thumb and fingers together in front of the other.
- Indicate that you could carry out the Rinne and Weber tests and examine the ears by auroscopy (see *Station 45*).

The glossopharyngeal nerve (CN IX)

- Indicate that you could test the gag reflex by touching the tonsillar fossae on both sides with an orange stick, but that this is likely to cause the patient some discomfort.

The vagus nerve (CN X)

- Ask the patient to phonate (say 'aah') and, aided by a pen flashlight, look for deviation of the uvula to the opposite side of the lesion. Use a tongue depressor if necessary.

The hypoglossal nerve (CN XII)

- Aided by a pen flashlight, inspect the tongue for wasting and fasciculation.
- Ask the patient to stick out his tongue and look for deviation to the side of the lesion. Now ask him to wiggle it from side to side.

The accessory nerve (CN XI)

- Look for wasting of the sternocleidomastoid and trapezius muscles.
- Ask the patient to:
  - shrug his shoulders against resistance
  - turn his head to either side against resistance

After the examination

- Thank the patient.
- Ensure that he is comfortable.
- If appropriate, state that you would order some key investigations, e.g. a CT or MRI.
- Summarize your findings and offer a differential diagnosis.

Conditions most likely to appear in a cranial nerve examination station

Third nerve palsy:

- the eye is depressed and abducted (down and out)
- elevation, adduction, and depression are limited, but abduction and intortion are normal
- there is a ptosis (drooping of the upper eyelid)
- the pupil may be dilated and unreactive to light or accommodation

Bell's (facial nerve) palsy:

- facial drooping and paralysis on the affected half
- if the forehead muscles are spared, it is a central rather than a peripheral palsy

Horner's syndrome:

- signs of Horner's syndrome are ptosis, miosis, enophthalmos, and facial anhidrosis

Cavernous sinus syndrome:

- the cavernous sinus contains the carotid artery and its sympathetic plexus, CN III, IV, and VI and the ophthalmic and maxillary branches of CN V
- signs of a cavernous sinus lesion may include (generally unilateral) proptosis, chemosis, ophthalmoplegia, and loss of sensation in the first and second divisions of the trigeminal nerve

Cerebellopontine angle syndrome:

- lesions in the area of the cerebellopontine angle can cause compression of CN V, VII, and VIII
- signs may include palsies of CN V and VII, nystagmus, ipsilateral deafness, and ipsilateral cerebellar signs

Bulbar palsy:

- lower motor neuron lesion in the medulla oblongata leads to bilateral impairment of function of CN IX–XII
- signs include speech difficulties, dysphagia, wasting and fasciculation of the tongue, absent palatal movements, absent gag reflex

Pseudo-bulbar palsy:

- upper motor neuron lesion in the corticobulbar pathways in the pyramidal tract leads to impairment of function of CN IX–XII and also CN V and VII
- signs include speech difficulties, dysphagia, conical and spastic tongue, brisk jaw jerk, emotional lability

Station 32

Motor system of the upper limbs examination

Before starting
- Introduce yourself to the patient.
- Explain the examination and ask for his permission to carry it out.
- Position him and ask him to expose his arms.
- Ask if he is currently experiencing any pain.

Junior Resident's tips

To recall the sequence of the peripheral neurological exam remember: 'To Postpone Reflexes Constitutes Stupidity' (Tone, Power, Reflexes, Coordination, Sensation)

The examination

Inspection
- Look for abnormal posturing.
- Look for abnormal movements such as tremor, fasciculation, dystonia, athetosis.
- Assess the muscles of the hands, arms, and shoulder girdle for size, shape, and symmetry. You can also measure the circumference of the arms.

Tone
- Ensure that the patient is not in any pain.
- Ask the patient to relax the muscles in his arms.
- Test the tone in the upper limbs by holding the patient's hand and simultaneously pronating and supinating and flexing and extending the forearm. If you suspect increased tone, ask the patient to clench his teeth and re-test. Is the increased tone best described as spasticity (clasp-knife) or as rigidity (lead pipe)? Spasticity suggests a pyramidal lesion, rigidity suggests an extra-pyramidal lesion.

Power
- Test muscle strength for shoulder abduction, elbow flexion and extension, wrist flexion and extension, finger flexion, extension, abduction and adduction, and thumb abduction and opposition. Compare muscle strength on both sides, and grade it on the MRC muscle strength scale:
  0 No movement.
  1 Feeble contractions.
  2 Movement, but not against gravity.
  3 Movement against gravity, but not against resistance.
  4 Movement against resistance, but not to full strength.
  5 Full strength.

Table 12. Important root values in the upper limb – muscle strength

• Shoulder abduction	C5
• Elbow flexion	C6
• Elbow extension	C7
• Wrist extension	C6, C7
• Wrist flexion	C7, C8
• Finger extension	C7 (radial nerve)
• Finger flexion	C8
• Finger abduction/adduction	T1 (ulnar nerve)
• Thumb abduction/opposition	T1 (median nerve)

Reflexes

- Test biceps, supinator, and triceps reflexes with a reflex hammer (see *Figure 34*). Compare both sides. If a reflex cannot be elicited, ask the patient to clench his teeth and re-test.

Table 13. Important root values in the upper limb – reflexes	
• Biceps	C5, C6
• Supinator	C6
• Triceps	C7

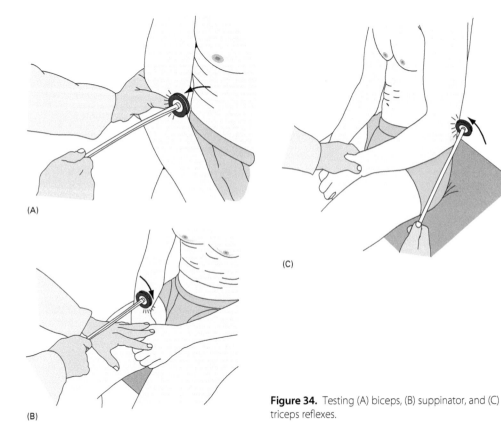

(A)

(C)

(B)

Figure 34. Testing (A) biceps, (B) suppinator, and (C) triceps reflexes.

Cerebellar signs

- Test for intention tremor, dysynergia, and dysmetria (past-pointing) by asking the patient to carry out the finger-to-nose test.
  - Place your index finger at about 2 feet from the patient's face. Ask him to touch the tip of his nose and then the tip of your finger with the tip of his index finger. Once he is able to do this, ask him to do it as fast as he can. And remember that he has two hands!
- Then test for dysdiadochokinesis.
  - Ask the patient to clap and then show him how to clap by alternating the palmar and dorsal surfaces of one hand. Once he is able to do this, ask him to do it as fast as he can. Ask him to repeat the test with his other hand.

After the examination

- Thank the patient.
- Ensure that he is comfortable.
- Ask to carry out a full neurological examination.
- In an exam, indicate that you would order some key investigations, e.g. CT, MRI, nerve conduction studies, electromyography, etc., if appropriate.
- Summarize your findings and offer a differential diagnosis.

Conditions most likely to come up in a motor system of the upper limbs examination

Parkinson's disease:
- motor signs include forward-flexed posture, mask-like facial expression, speech difficulties, resting tremor, cogwheel rigidity, bradykinesia

Cerebellar lesion:
- motor signs depend on the anatomy of the lesion, and may include nystagmus, slurred or staccato speech, hypotonia, hyporeflexia, intention tremor, dysmetria, dysynergia, dysdiadochokinesis, ataxia

Ulnar nerve lesion:
- wasting, weakness, numbness, and tingling in the fifth finger and in the medial half of the fourth finger
- curling up of the fifth and fourth fingers ('ulnar claw') indicates that the nerve is severely affected

Median nerve lesion:
- a lesion at the level of the wrist produces wasting of the thenar muscles, weakness of abduction and opposition of the thumb, and numbness over the palmar aspect of the thumb, index finger, third finger, and lateral half of the fourth finger
- a lesion at the level of the forearm produces additional weakness of flexion of the distal and middle phalanges
- a lesion at the level of the elbow or above produces additional weakness of pronation of the forearm and ulnar deviation of the wrist on wrist flexion

Radial nerve lesion:
- a lesion at the level of the axilla or above produces weakness of elbow extension and flexion, weakness of wrist and finger extension with attending wrist drop and finger drop, weakness of thumb abduction and extension, and sensory loss over the dorsoradial aspect of the hand and the dorsal aspect of the radial 3½ fingers (usually circumscribed to a small, triangular area over the first dorsal web space)
- inferior lesions are likely to spare triceps (elbow extension), brachioradialis (elbow flexion), and extensor carpi radialis longus (wrist extension and radial abduction, but only one of five wrist extensors)

Radiculopathy, affecting a single root nerve (see *Table 13*)

Hemiplegia/hemiparesis:
- paralysis or weakness on one side of the body accompanied by decreased movement control, spasticity, and hyper-reflexia (upper motor neuron syndrome)

Myopathy:
- symmetrical weakness predominantly affecting proximal muscle groups
- in contrast to neuropathy, in myopathy muscle atrophy and hyporeflexia occur very late

Sensory system of the upper limbs examination

Before starting

- Introduce yourself to the patient.
- Explain the examination and ask for his permission to carry it out.
- Position him so that he is comfortably seated and ask him to expose his arms and to position them so that the palms are facing towards you.
- Ask if he is currently experiencing any pain.

The examination

To examine the sensory system, test light touch, pain, vibration sense, and proprioception.

 Do not forget to inspect the arms before you start. In particular, look for muscle wasting, fasciculation, scars and other obvious signs.

- Light touch (not light rub). Ask the patient to close his eyes and to say 'yes' each time he is touched with a wisp of cotton wool. Apply the cotton wool to his sternum as a test. Then apply it to each of the dermatomes of the arm, moving from the hand and up along the arm. Remember to compare both sides as you go along.
- Pain. Ask the patient to close his eyes and apply a sharp object – ideally a neurological pin – to the sternum and then to each of the dermatomes of the arm, as above. Compare both sides as you go along. If there is any loss of or difference in sensation, map out the area affected.

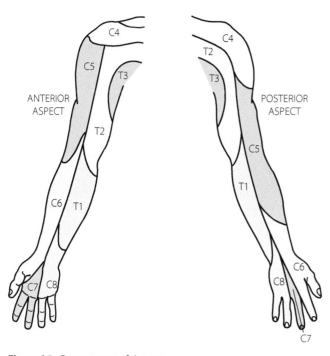

Figure 35. Dermatomes of the arm.

- Vibration. Ask the patient to close his eyes and apply a vibrating 128 Hz or 256 Hz tuning fork (not the smaller 512 Hz tuning fork used in hearing tests) to the sternum and then over the bony prominences of the arm, starting with the interphalangeal joint of the thumb and moving up to the wrist and then the elbow. Compare both sides as you go along.
- Proprioception. Ensure that the patient does not suffer from arthritis or from some other painful condition of the hand. Ask him to close his eyes. Hold the distal interphalangeal joint of his index finger between the thumb and index finger of one hand. With the other hand, move the distal phalanx up and down at the joint, asking him to identify the direction of each movement, e.g. *"I'm going to move your finger up and down. Is this up or down?" "What about this? And that?"* Compare both sides.

After the examination

- Thank the patient.
- Ensure that he is comfortable.
- Ask to carry out a full neurological examination.
- In an exam, summarize your findings and offer a differential diagnosis.

Conditions most likely to come up in a sensory examination of the upper limbs station
Mononeuropathy:
• lesion affecting a single nerve, e.g. ulnar, median, or radial nerve (see *Station 32*)
Polyneuropathy:
• lesion affecting multiple nerves in a glove and stocking distribution, such as in diabetic neuropathy
Radiculopathy:
• lesion affecting a single root nerve, e.g. C6
Brown–Séquard syndrome:
• numbness to touch and vibration and loss of proprioception (and weakness) on same side of the lesion, and loss of pain and temperature sensation on the opposite side
• caused by lateral hemisection or injury of the spinal cord
Syringomyelia:
• loss of pain and temperature sensation but not of other sensory modalities

Motor system of the lower limbs examination

Before starting

- Introduce yourself to the patient.
- Explain the examination and ask for his permission to carry it out.
- Position him and ask him to expose his legs.
- Ask if he is currently experiencing any pain.

The examination

Inspection

- Look for deformities of the foot.
- Look for abnormal posturing.
- Look for fasciculation.
- Assess the muscles of the legs for size, shape, and symmetry. You can also measure the circumference of the quadriceps or calves.

Tone

- Ensure that the patient is not in any pain.
- Ask the patient to relax the muscles in his legs.
- Test the tone in the legs by rolling the leg on the bed, by flexing and extending the knee, and/or by abruptly lifting the leg at the knee.

Power

- Test muscle strength for hip flexion, extension, abduction and adduction, knee flexion and extension, plantar flexion and dorsiflexion of the foot and big toe, and inversion and eversion of the forefoot. Compare muscle strength on both sides, and grade it on the MRC scale for muscle strength:
  - **0** No movement.
  - **1** Feeble contractions.
  - **2** Movement, but not against gravity.
  - **3** Movement against gravity, but not against resistance.
  - **4** Movement against resistance, but not to full strength.
  - **5** Full strength.

Table 14. Important root values in the lower limb – muscle strength	
• Hip flexion	L1, L2
• Hip extension	S1
• Hip adduction	L2
• Knee flexion	L5, S1
• Knee extension	L3, L4
• Foot dorsiflexion	L4, L5
• Foot plantar flexion	S1
• Big toe dorsiflexion	L5

Reflexes

- Test the knee jerk and ankle jerk with a reflex hammer (see *Figure 36*). Test the knee jerk by raising and supporting the knee with one arm and striking the patellar tendon with the other. To test the ankle jerk, abduct and externally rotate the hip and flex the knee and ankle. Then strike at the Achilles tendon. Compare both sides. If a reflex cannot be elicited, ask the patient to clench his teeth and re-test.

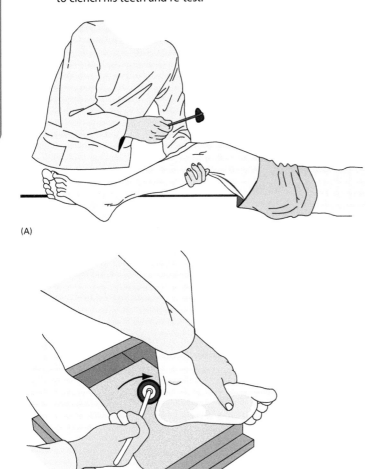

(A)

(B)

Figure 36. Testing the knee (A) and ankle (B) reflexes.

- Test for clonus by holding up the ankle and rapidly dorsiflexing the foot.
- Test for the Babinsky sign (extensor plantar reflex) by scraping the side of the foot with the sharp end of a reflex hammer. The sign is positive if there is extension of the big toe at the MTP joint, so-called 'upgoing plantars'.

Table 15. Important root values in the lower limb – reflexes	
Knee jerk	L3, L4
Ankle jerk	S1

Cerebellar signs

- Carry out the heel-to-shin test.
  - Lie the patient on an exam table. Ask him to run the heel of one leg down the shin of the other, and then to bring the heel back up to the knee and to start again. Ask him to repeat the test with his other leg.

Gait

- If he can, ask the patient to walk to the end of the room and to turn around and walk back. (See *Station 36: Gait, co-ordination, and cerebellar function examination*.)

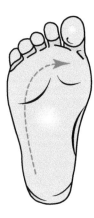

Figure 37. Testing for the Babinsky or extensor plantar sign.

After the examination

- Thank the patient.
- Ensure that he is comfortable.
- Ask to carry out a full neurological examination.
- In an exam, indicate that you would order some key investigations, e.g. CT, MRI, nerve conduction studies, electromyography, etc., if appropriate.
- Summarize your findings and offer a differential diagnosis.

Conditions most likely to come up in a motor system of the lower limbs examination station	
Mononeuropathy: • lesion affecting a single nerve, most commonly the common peroneal nerve (resulting in foot drop)	**Cauda equina lesion:** • signs include unilateral or bilateral lower limb motor and/or sensory deficits • the ankle jerks are usually absent on both sides • upper motor neuron signs such as Babinsky sign and clonus are absent
Polyneuropathy: • lesion affecting multiple nerves in a glove and stocking distribution as in diabetic neuropathy	
Radiculopathy: • lesion affecting a single root nerve (see *Table 15*)	**Myopathy:** • symmetrical weakness predominantly affecting proximal muscle groups • in contrast to neuropathy, in myopathy muscle atrophy and hyporeflexia occur very late
Hemiplegia/hemiparesis: • paralysis or weakness on one side of the body accompanied by decreased movement control, spasticity, and hyperreflexia (upper motor neuron syndrome)	

Station 35

Sensory system of the lower limbs examination

Before starting

- Introduce yourself to the patient.
- Explain the examination and ask for his permission to carry it out.
- Position him on an exam table and ask him to expose his legs.
- Ask if he is currently experiencing any pain.

The examination

To examine the sensory system, test light touch, pain, vibration sense, and proprioception.

- Do not forget to inspect the legs before you start. In particular, look for muscle wasting, fasciculation, scars, and any other obvious signs.
- Light touch (not light rub). Ask the patient to close his eyes and to say 'yes' each time he is touched with a wisp of cotton wool. Apply the cotton wool to his sternum as a test. Then apply it to each of the dermatomes of the leg, moving from the foot and up along the leg. Remember to compare both sides as you go along.
- Pain. Ask the patient to close his eyes and apply a sharp object – ideally a neurological pin – to the sternum and then to each of the dermatomes of the leg, as above. Compare both sides as you go along. If there is any loss of or difference in sensation, map out the area affected.
- Vibration. Ask the patient to close his eyes and apply a vibrating 128 Hz or 256 Hz tuning fork (not the smaller 512 Hz tuning fork used in hearing tests) to the sternum and then over the bony prominences of the leg, starting with the interphalangeal joint of the big toe. Compare both sides as you go along.

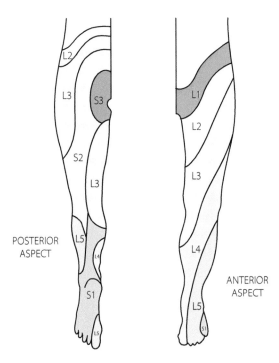

Figure 38. Dermatomes of the leg.

- Proprioception. Ensure that the patient does not suffer from arthritis, gout, or some other painful condition of the foot. Ask him to close his eyes. Hold the interphalangeal joint of his big toe between the thumb and index finger of one hand. With the other hand, move the distal phalanx up and down at the joint, asking him to identify the direction of each movement, e.g. *"I'm going to move your toe up and down. Is this up or down?" "What about this? And that?"* Compare both sides. If the patient is able to stand, you can also perform Romberg's test (see *Station 36: Gait, co-ordination, and cerebellar function examination*).

After the examination

- Thank the patient.
- Ensure that he is comfortable.
- Ask to carry out a full neurological examination.
- In an exam, indicate that you would order some key investigations, e.g. CT, MRI, nerve conduction studies, electromyography, etc., if appropriate.
- Summarize your findings and offer a differential diagnosis.

Conditions most likely to come up in a sensory system of the lower limbs examination station
Mononeuropathy:
• lesion affecting a single nerve
Polyneuropathy:
• lesion affecting multiple nerves as in alcoholic or diabetic neuropathy
Radiculopathy:
• lesion affecting a single root nerve (see *Figure 38*)
Cauda equina lesion:
• signs include unilateral or bilateral lower limb motor and/or sensory deficits, including 'saddle anesthesia' (loss of sensation in the area of the buttocks and perineum)
Hemisensory loss:
• loss of sensation including light, pain, temperature, vibration, and proprioception on one side of the body
• normally accompanied by hemiplegia/hemiparesis with attendant spasticity and hyper-reflexia (upper motor neuron syndrome)
Brown–Séquard syndrome:
• numbness to touch and vibration and loss of proprioception (and weakness) on same side of the lesion, and loss of pain and temperature sensation on the opposite side
• caused by lateral hemisection or injury of the spinal cord
Posterior column disease:
• loss of proprioception and vibration but not of other sensory modalities

Gait, co-ordination, and cerebellar function examination

Before starting

- Introduce yourself to the patient.
- Explain the examination and ask for his consent to carry it out.
- Ask if he is currently experiencing any pain.

Examination of gait

- Inspection. Inspect the patient in the sitting position, noting any abnormalities of posture. Ask him to stand up and ensure that he is steady on his feet. Truncal ataxis suggests a midline cerebellar lesion. Inspect posture from both front and side.
- Gait and arm swing. Ask him to walk to the end of the room and to turn around and walk back. If he normally uses a stick or walker, he should not be prevented from doing so. Note the gait and also the arm swing and any difficulty in standing or turning.
- Heel-to-toe test. Ask him to walk heel-to-toe, 'as if on a tightrope'. Ataxia on a narrow-based gait suggests a cerebellar or vestibular lesion.
- Romberg's test. Ask him to stand unaided with his feet together, his arms by his sides and his eyes closed. If he sways and threatens to lose his balance, the test is said to be positive, indicating posterior column disease.

 You must be in a position to steady the patient should he appear to fall.

Examination of co-ordination

- Resting tremor. Ask the patient to sit down, to rest his hands in his lap, and to close his eyes. Resting tremor is a sign of Parkinson's disease.
- Intention tremor. Ask the patient to do something, e.g. remove his watch or write a sentence.
- Muscle tone in the arms. Examine muscle tone in the elbow (flexion and extension) and wrist (flexion and extension, abduction and adduction) joints. Compare both sides.
- Dysdiadochokinesis. Ask the patient to clap and then show him how to clap by alternating the palmar and dorsal surfaces of one hand. Once he is able to do this, ask him to do it as fast as he can. Ask him to repeat the test with his other hand.
- Finger-to-nose test. Place your index finger at about 2 feet from the patient's face. Ask him to touch the tip of his nose and then the tip of your finger with the tip of his index finger. Once he is able to do this, ask him to do it as fast as he can. And remember that he has two hands! Look for intention tremor and dysmetria (past-pointing), both signs of cerebellar disease.
- Fine finger movements. Ask the patient to oppose his thumb with each of his other fingers in turn. Once he is able to do this, ask him to do it as fast as he can. Again, remember that he has two hands.
- Muscle tone in the legs. Ask the patient to lie down on the exam table and, if possible, to relax the muscles in his legs. Test the tone in his legs by rolling the leg on the bed, by flexing and extending the knee, and/or by abruptly lifting the leg at the knee.
- Heel-to-shin test. Ask the patient to run the heel of one leg down the shin of the other, and then to bring the heel back up to the knee and to start again. Ask him to repeat the test with his other leg.

Assessment of cerebellar function

- If you need to assess cerebellar function, specifically, carry out the above plus test eye movements (nystagmus) and ask the patient to say 'baby hippopotamus' (slurred/staccato speech). If you are then asked to list cerebellar signs, simply remember the acronym DANISH:
  - **D**ysdiadochokinesis and dysmetria (finger overshoot)
  - **A**taxia
  - **N**ystagmus – test eye movements
  - **I**ntention tremor
  - **S**lurred/staccato speech – ask the patient to say 'baby hippopotamus' or 'British constitution'
  - **H**ypotonia/hyporeflexia

After the examination

- Ask the patient if he has any questions or concerns.
- Thank the patient.
- Ensure that he is comfortable.
- Ask to carry out a full neurological examination.
- Summarize your findings and offer a differential diagnosis.

Conditions most likely to come up in a gait and co-ordination examination
Hemiplegic gait:
• the pelvis tilts upward, the hip is abducted, and the leg is swung forward in a semi-circular movement
• the leg is stiff and extended but the arm may be held in flexion and adduction with minimal swing
Scissor gait:
• a spastic gait seen in cerebral palsy and resulting from muscle contractures
• the hips, knees, and ankles are flexed, producing a crouching and tiptoeing appearance
• in addition, the hips are adducted and internally rotated, such that the knees cross or hit each other in a scissor-like movement
Festinating gait:
• seen in Parkinson's disease
• short shuffling steps with stiff arms and legs and stooped posture; difficulty starting and turning
Ataxic gait:
• seen in spinal and cerebellar lesions and in alcohol intoxication
• unsteady, broad-based gait with a lurching quality
Neuropathic gait:
• seen in peripheral neuropathies
• weak foot dorsiflexors result in a high-stepping gait with foot-slapping; the high-stepping is an attempt to prevent the foot from dragging and being injured; also called 'high-stepping gait' or 'foot-slapping gait'

Trendelenburg gait:

- seen in weakness of the hip abductors or in an inability or reluctance to abduct the hip, e.g. due to a fractured neck of femur or to arthritic pain
- the pelvis tilts to the unaffected side in the stance phase; as a result, the trunk lurches to the affected side in an attempt to maintain a level pelvis
- bilateral Trendelenburg results in a typical waddling gait

Antalgic gait:

- seen in arthritis and trauma
- avoidance of motions that trigger pain
- often quick, short, and light footsteps
- not to be confused with a Trendelenburg gait

Myopathic gait:

- in muscular diseases the proximal pelvic girdle muscles are most affected, such that the patient is unable to stabilize the pelvis in the stance phase
- the pelvis drops to the side of the leg being raised, and this results in a broad-based, waddling gait

Speech assessment

The patient is likely to find the assessment difficult and distressing, so remember to be especially empathetic. In particular, do not rush the examination or keep on interrupting the patient, but move at a pace that feels comfortable for him.

Table 16. Definitions	
Dysphonia	Impairment of ability to vocalize speech.
Dysarthria	Impairment of ability to articulate speech.
Dysphasia	Impairment of ability to comprehend or express language.
Expressive dysphasia (Broca's area, in the inferolateral dominant frontal lobe) and receptive dysphasia (Wernicke's area, in the posterior superior dominant temporal lobe) often co-exist.	

Before starting

- Introduce yourself to the patient.
- Explain the assessment and obtain his consent to carry it out.
- Ask him to try to describe his current problems.

The assessment

Orientation in time and place

Time

Name: (year) (season) (month) (date) (day)

Place

Name: (country) (state/region) (city) (hospital) (floor)

Dysphasia

Expressive

Assess whether the patient has difficulty in finding the right words whilst in conversation with you.

Nominal

Ask the patient to name some common objects such as a watch, pen, or dime; then to name the components of some of these objects, e.g. hour hand, winder, strap. Note that nominal dysphasia is a common form of expressive dysphasia.

Receptive

Assess whether the patient has difficulty understanding you by asking him to carry out some simple instructions such as 'shut your eyes', 'touch your nose', and 'point to the door'.

Dysarthria

Ask the patient to repeat some of the following: 'British constitution', 'West Register Street', 'Baby hippopotamus', 'Biblical criticism', and 'Artillery'.

Assess the structures involved in phonation and articulation by asking the patient to repeat:

- 'Me, me, me'   Lips
- 'La, la, la'   Tongue
- 'Khu, gut'   Palate
- 'Ah'   Palate, larynx, and expiratory muscles

Dysphonia

- Make a note of the patient's volume of speech, which may be low if there is weakness of the vocal cords or respiratory muscles. Ask the patient to cough, and look out for 'bovine' cough.

Dyslexia

- Correct the patient's vision and ask him to read a short paragraph from a newspaper or magazine, and bear in mind the patient's level of education and likely reading level.

Dyscalculia

- Ask the patient to carry out simple sums and subtractions.

Dysgraphia

- Ask the patient to write a sentence.

After the assessment

- Ask the patient if he has any questions or concerns.
- Thank the patient.
- Summarize your findings, offer a differential diagnosis, and state the probable area of the lesion.

Conditions most likely to come up in a speech assessment station

Dsyphasia:

- expressive dysphasia results from damage to Broca's area in the left inferior frontal region
- there is 'telegraphic speech' characterized by reduction in word range and non-fluent speech with errors of grammar and syntax
- receptive dysphasia results from damage to Wernicke's area in the left superior posterior temporal lobe
- comprehension is poor and speech, although fluent, may be meaningless
- global dysphasia results from damage to both Broca's area and Wernicke's area
- there is both poor comprehension and lack of fluency

Dysarthria (slurred speech):

- can result from lesions of the tongue, lips, or mouth; bilateral upper motor neuron lesions of the corticobulbar tract (pseudobulbar or spastic dysarthria, 'hot potato speech'); bulbar palsy (nasal speech with slurring of labial and lingual consonants); cerebellar lesions (scanning or staccato speech); Parkinson's disease (monotonous speech with a soft voice); or myasthenia gravis (nasal speech with hoarseness and vocal fatigue), amongst others

Dysphonia:

- results from vocal cord pathology, as in laryngitis, or from damage to the vagal nerve supply to the vocal cords
- bovine cough results from inability to abduct vocal cords

Dyslexia, dyscalculia, dysgraphia:

- result from lesions of the dominant parietal lobe

Station 38

General psychiatric history

Specifications: In an exam, the instructions are likely to ask you to focus on the chief psychiatric complaint.

 In taking a psychiatric history, it is especially important to put the patient at ease and to be seen to be sensitive, tactful, and empathetic.

Before starting

- Introduce yourself to the patient.
- Ensure that he is comfortable. Make some general comments to put him at ease and build a rapport.

The history

- Name, age, and mode of referral (if not already provided).

Chief complaint and history of presenting illness

- Ask mainly open questions, e.g. *Can you tell me why you've come to the hospital today?* Try to form a diagnostic hypothesis and to validate or falsify it by asking further questions (logico-deductive approach).
- Ask about:
  - the onset and duration of symptoms
  - the effect the symptoms are having on the patient's everyday life
  - any treatments so far
- If you have not done so already, ask screening questions about mood, anxiety, obsessions, abnormal beliefs, and abnormal perceptions (see *Station 39: Mental state examination*).

Past psychiatric history

- Previous episodes of illness.
- Previous treatments and their outcomes.
- Previous admissions, formal and informal.
- History of neglect or self-harm.
- History of violence.

Past medical history

- Current illness:
  - acute illness
  - chronic illness
  - vascular risk factors
- Past and childhood illnesses, including head injury.
- Surgery.

Drug history/current treatments

- Psychological treatments.
- Prescribed medication.

- Recent changes in prescribed medication.
- Over-the-counter drugs.
- Allergies.

Substance use

- Alcohol.
- Tobacco.
- Illicit drugs.

[Note]   Further questioning to establish dependence may be required if alcohol use and/or illicit drug use is high (see *Station 42: Alcohol history*).

Family history

- Determine if anyone in the family has suffered from psychiatric illness or attempted suicide, e.g. *"Has anyone in the family ever had a nervous breakdown?"*
- Partner: age or age at death, occupation, health.
- Children: age or age at death, occupation, health.
- Quality of relationships and atmosphere in the home.
- Recent events in the family.

Social history

- Self-care.
- Social support.
- Housing.
- Finances.
- Typical day.
- Interests and hobbies.
- Predominant mood and premorbid personality.

Personal history

- Birth.
- Developmental milestones.
- Childhood: emotional problems, serious illnesses, prolonged separation from parents.
- Educational achievement.
- Occupational history.
- Forensic history.
- Psychosexual history: past and present partners (including same sex partners), quality of relationships, frequency of sexual intercourse, sexual problems, physical or sexual abuse.
- Forensic history, e.g. *"Have you ever had problems with the police or with the law?"*
- Religious or spiritual orientation, e.g. *"Do you believe there is something beyond us, like God?"*

After taking the history

- Ask the patient if there is anything he might add that you have forgotten to ask about.
- Indicate that you could check the patient's psychiatric records (if any) and take an informant history, for example, from a relative, friend, caregiver, police officer, family doctor, or other healthcare professional.
- Summarize your findings and offer a differential diagnosis.
- Thank the patient.

Common conditions most likely to appear in a psychiatric history station

- Depressive disorder
- Anxiety disorder, e.g. agoraphobia, social phobia, panic disorder, generalized anxiety disorder
- Mixed depression–anxiety
- Obsessive–compulsive disorder
- Eating disorder
- Mania and bipolar affective disorder
- Schizophrenia and other delusional disorders

NB. For descriptions of these conditions, see *Table 17* at the end of *Station 39*.

Mental state examination

Specifications: In an exam, you may be asked to perform the mental state exam as part of a wider assessment or you may be asked to focus on only one part of the mental state assessment.

Before starting

- Introduce yourself to the patient.
- Explain that you would like to explore his thoughts and feelings, and ask him if this is OK.
- Take out a pen and pad.

Assessing the mental state

The mental state can be assessed under 7 main headings:
1. Appearance and behavior.
2. Speech.
3. Mood.
4. Abnormal thoughts.
5. Abnormal experiences.
6. Cognition.
7. Insight.

Appearance and behavior

Begin by asking the patient some open questions, and focusing your attention on his *appearance and behavior*.

- Level of consciousness.
- Appearance: body build, posture, general physical condition, grooming and hygiene, dress, physical stigmata such as scars, piercings, and tattoos.
- Inappropriate behavior and attitude to the examiner. In particular note: facial expression, degree of eye contact, and quality of rapport.
- Motor activity/disorders of movement, e.g. agitation, retardation, tremor, dystonias, mannerisms.

Speech

Note:

- Amount, rate, volume, and tone of speech, e.g. logorrhea (large amount of speech), pressure of speech (increased rate of speech), poverty of speech (small amount of speech), speech retardation (decreased rate of speech), mutism (no speech).
- Form of speech, e.g. circumstantiality, tangentiality, clang associations, puns, rhymes, neologisms, perseverations. In circumstantiality, speech is organized and goal-oriented but cramped by excessive or irrelevant detail and parenthetical remarks. In tangentiality, speech is organized but not goal-oriented in that it is only very indirectly related to the questions being asked.

Mood

Note or ask about:

- Current mood state and severity. If there is the suggestion of depression, ask the patient to rate his mood on a scale of 1 to 10, with 1 being the worst that he has ever felt and 10 being normal.

Clinical Skills for Medical Students

- Biological symptoms: sleep, appetite, libido, energy.
- Ideas of harm to self, e.g. *"People with problems similar to those that you have been describing often feel that life is no longer worth living. Have you felt that life is no longer worth living?"* If yes, then this should be explored further: *"Have you ever thought of killing yourself?" "Have you made any plans?" "Would you carry out those plans?" "What stops/would stop you?"*.
- Ideas of harm to others.
- Anxiety and anxiety symptoms, e.g. butterflies, giddiness, clamminess, palpitations, difficulty catching breath. If there is the suggestion of an anxiety disorder, this should be explored further.

 In an exam, you are likely to fail this station if you do not ask about ideas of harm in an at-risk patient.

Abnormal thoughts

Note or ask about:

- Stream of thought, e.g. pressure of thought, poverty of thought, thought blocking.
- Form of thought, e.g. flight of ideas, loosening of associations, over-inclusive thinking.
- Content of thought.
  - Preoccupations, ruminations, obsessions, and compulsive acts, e.g. for obsessions, *"Do certain things keep coming into your mind even though you try hard to keep them out?"* And for compulsive acts, *"Do you ever find yourself spending a lot of time doing the same thing over and over again even though you've already done it well enough?"*
  - Phobias, e.g. *"Do you have any special fears, like some people are afraid of spiders or snakes?"*
  - Delusions and overvalued ideas. For obvious reasons, you cannot easily ask directly about delusions. Begin by an introductory statement and general questions, such as *"I would like to ask you some questions that might seem a little bit strange. These are questions that we ask to everyone who comes to see us. Is that all right with you? Do you have any ideas that your friends and family do not share?"* Explore any delusions and in particular ask about their onset, their effect on the patient's life, and the patient's explanation for them (degree of insight). If necessary, ask specifically about common delusional themes, e.g. delusions of persecution, reference, control, guilt, grandeur.

Abnormal experiences

Ask about:

- Illusions and hallucinations. Again begin by an introductory statement and general questions, such as *"I gather that you have been under quite some pressure recently. When people are under pressure they sometimes find that their imagination plays tricks on them. Have you had any such experiences? Have you seen things which other people cannot see? Have you heard things which other people cannot hear?"* Ask about all five modalities and explore any positive findings for content, onset, frequency, duration, and effect on the patient's life. Exclude pseudohallucinations and hypnogogic and hypnopompic hallucinations. For auditory hallucinations of voices, determine if there is more than one voice, and if the voices talk to the patient (second person) or about him (third person). If the voices talk to him, do they command him to do dangerous things and, importantly, is he likely to act on these commands? If the voices talk about him, do they comment on his every thought and action (running commentary)? Other forms of auditory hallucinations are *écho de la pensée* and *gedankenlautwerden*, both first rank symptoms of schizophrenia.

Junior Resident's tips

Echo de la pensée refers to the phenomenon where the patient hears his thoughts echoed by an external voice.

Gedankenlautwerden literally means 'thoughts becoming loud' and refers to a hallucination where the patient hears voices that anticipate what he is about to think.

Differentiating between true hallucinations and pseudo-hallucinations

A pseudo-hallucination may differ from a true hallucination in that:

- it is perceived to arise from the mind (inner space) rather than the sense organs (outer space)
- it is less vivid
- it is less distressing
- the patient may have some degree of control over it

True hallucinations tend to be a feature of functional disorders, whereas pseudo-hallucinations tend to be a feature of personality disorder. This is, however, not a hard and fast rule.

- Depersonalization and derealization, e.g. for depersonalization *'Have you ever felt unreal?'* And for derealization, *'Have you ever felt that things around you are unreal?'*

Cognition

Generally speaking, a quick and informal cognitive assessment can be carried out by recording the following:

- Orientation in time, place, and person
- Attention and concentration, e.g. serial sevens test, spelling 'world' backward. Record the time taken and the number of errors
- Memory:
  - short-term memory: ask the patient to name and remember three objects, then carry out the serial sevens test, then ask him to recall the three objects
  - recent memory: ask him how he came to the clinic this morning/afternoon
  - remote memory: ask him where he was born, where he grew up, etc.
- Grasp: ask the patient to name the current president and vice-president.

If cognitive impairment is suspected, you can carry out the Folstein Mini-Mental State Examination (MMSE). The MMSE is scored out of 30. Scores of less than 22 are indicative of significant cognitive impairment, while scores of 22 to 25 are indicative of moderate cognitive impairment. The result is invalid if the patient is delirious or has an affective disorder.

Insight

To determine degree of insight, ask the patient:

- *"Do you think there is anything wrong with you?"*

If no,

- *"Why did you come to hospital?"*

If yes,

- *"What do you think is wrong with you?"*
- *"What do you think the cause of it is?"*
- *"Do you think you need treatment?"*
- *"What are you hoping treatment will do for you?"*

After the mental state examination

- Thank the patient.
- Ensure that he is comfortable.
- Summarize your findings. Note that mood should be reported as subjective mood and objective mood. Do not omit to comment upon risk.
- Offer a differential diagnosis.

Table 17. Principal features of key psychiatric disorders
See ICD-10 or DSM-IV for detailed diagnostic criteria.

Depressive disorder	See *Station 40*
Mania	• Garish clothing, accessories, and makeup • Hyperactive, flirtatious, hypervigilant, assertive, and/or aggressive behavior • Pressured speech; abnormalities of the form of speech • Euphoric or irritable or labile mood • Grandiose thoughts with flight of ideas and loosening of associations; mood congruent delusions • Hallucinations • Poor concentration • Poor insight
Schizophrenia	• Delusions • Hallucinations • Disorganized speech • Disorganized or catatonic behaviour • Negative symptoms
Agoraphobia	Persistent irrational fear of places difficult or embarrassing to escape from, such as places that are confined, crowded, or far from home. Increased reliance on trusted companions for accompaniment or, in severe cases, restriction to the home.
Social phobia	Persistent irrational fear of being scrutinized by others and of being embarrassed or humiliated, either in most social situations or in specific social situations such as public speaking.
Specific phobia	Persistent irrational fear of one or more objects or situations. Common specific phobias include heights, darkness, enclosed spaces, storms, animals, flying, driving, blood, injections, and dental and medical procedures.
Panic disorder	Panic attacks are characterized by rapid onset of severe anxiety lasting for about 20–30 minutes. They may occur in the phobic anxiety disorder listed above or in other disorders such as OCD, PTSD, and organic disorders. In panic disorder, panic attacks occur recurrently and unexpectedly. There is fear of the implications and consequences of an attack, e.g. having a heart attack, losing control, 'going crazy'. Anticipatory fear of panic attacks develops and may itself lead to further panic attacks and to significant behavioral changes such as the development of agoraphobia.

continued

Psychiatry

Table 17. Principal features of key psychiatric disorders – *continued*

Generalized anxiety disorder	Long-standing free-floating anxiety that may fluctuate but that is neither situational (phobic anxiety disorders) nor episodic (panic disorder). There is apprehension about a number of events far out of proportion to the actual likelihood or impact of the feared events. Other common symptoms include symptoms of autonomic arousal, irritability, poor concentration, muscle tension, tiredness, and sleep disturbances.
Obsessive compulsive disorder (OCD)	An obsessional thought is a recurrent idea, image, or impulse that is perceived as being senseless, that is unsuccessfully resisted, and that results in marked anxiety and distress.
	A compulsive act is a recurrent stereotyped behavior that is not useful or enjoyable but that reduces anxiety and distress. It is usually perceived as being senseless and is unsuccessfully resisted. A compulsive act may be a response to an obsessive thought or according to rules that must be applied rigidly.
Post-traumatic stress disorder (PTSD)	A protracted and sometimes delayed response to a highly threatening or catastrophic experience characterized by numbing, detachment, flashbacks, nightmares, partial or complete amnesia for the event, avoidance of (and distress at) reminders of the event, and prominent anxiety symptoms. Associated psychiatric disorders are very common, especially depressive disorders, anxiety disorders, and alcohol and substance misuse.
Adjustment disorder	A protracted response to a significant life change or life event characterized by depressive symptoms and/or anxiety symptoms that are not severe enough to meet a diagnosis of depressive disorder or anxiety disorder, but that nevertheless lead to an impairment of social functioning.
Somatization disorder (Briquet's syndrome)	A long history of multiple and severe physical symptoms that cannot be accounted for by a physical disorder or other psychiatric disorder. Compare to factitious disorders such as Münchausen syndrome and to malingering.
Hypochondriacal disorder (hypochondriasis)	A fear or belief of having a serious physical disorder despite medical reassurance to the contrary.
Eating disorders	See *Station 43*.
Alcohol dependence	See *Station 42*.

Depression history

 For this chief complaint, it is especially important to put the patient at ease and to be sensitive, tactful, and empathetic.

Before starting

- Introduce yourself to the patient.
- Explain that you are going to ask him some questions about his feelings, and ask for his consent to do this.
- Ensure that he is comfortable.
- Unless this information has been provided, ask for his name, age, and occupation.

The interview

- First ask open questions about the patient's current mood, listening attentively and gently encouraging him to open up.
- Ask about the onset of illness, and about its triggers and causes.

Ensure that you ask about:

- The core features of depression:
  - depressed mood
  - loss of interest
  - fatiguability
- Other common features of depression:
  - poor concentration
  - poor self-esteem and self-confidence
  - guilt
  - pessimism/hopelessness
- The somatic features of depression:
  - sleep disturbance
  - early morning waking
  - morning depression
  - loss of appetite and/or weight loss
  - loss of libido
  - anhedonia
  - agitation and/or retardation
- Screen for possible anxiety, hallucinations, delusions, and mania, so as to exclude other possible psychiatric diagnoses.
- Take brief past medical, drug, family, and social history. Remember that drugs and alcohol are a common cause of depression.
- Assess the severity of the illness and its effect on the patient's life.

 Ask about suicidal ideation (also see Station 41: Suicide risk assessment). *In an exam, you may fail this station if you don't!*

> **Asking about suicidal ideation**
>
> Asking about suicide can feel uncomfortable for some. Use a formulation such as, *"People with problems similar to those that you have been describing often feel that life is no longer worth living. Have you felt that life is no longer worth living?"* If yes, then this should be explored further: *"Have you ever thought of killing yourself?" "Have you made any plans?" "Would you carry out those plans?" "What stops/ would stop you?"*

After finishing

- Ask the patient if there is anything he might add that you have forgotten to ask about.
- Thank him.
- Summarize your findings and suggest a further course of action, for example, further assessment of suicidal risk (see *Station 41*), follow-up by the acute psychiatry service, or, admission to a psychiatric unit.

Suicide risk assessment

And so it was I entered the broken world
To trace the visionary company of love, its voice
An instant in the wind (I know not whither hurled)
But not for long to hold each desperate choice.

From *Broken Tower*, by Hart Crane (b. 1899; d. 1932, by suicide)

Before starting

- Introduce yourself to the patient.
- Establish rapport.

The assessment

Ask about:

- The history of the current episode of self-harm (if any) to determine degree of suicidal intent (higher intent/lower intent – guidelines only):
  - what was the precipitant for the attempt? (serious precipitant/trivial precipitant)
  - was it planned? (planned/unplanned)
  - what was the method of self-harm, and did he expect this to be lethal? (violent method/ non-violent method)
  - did he make a will or leave a suicide note? (suicide note/no suicide note)
  - was he alone? (alone/not alone)
  - did he take any precautions against discovery? (precautions/no precautions)
  - was he intoxicated?
  - did he seek help after the attempt? (sought help/did not seek help)
  - how did he feel when help arrived? (angry or disappointed/relieved)
- Assess risk factors for suicide:
  - previous suicide attempt(s)
  - recent life crisis
  - male sex, especially if between the ages of 25 and 44
  - divorced, widowed, or single
  - unemployed or in certain occupations, e.g. medicine, farming
  - poor level of social support
  - physical illness
  - psychiatric illness
  - substance misuse
  - family history of depression, substance misuse, or suicide
- Mental state: assess current mood and exclude psychosis.
- Will he be returning to the same situation? What has changed? Are there any important protective factors?
- Ask about current suicidal ideation. Has he made any plans?

After the assessment

- Thank the patient.
- Summarize your findings, state the patient's suicide risk, and suggest a plan of action (e.g. further investigations, psychiatric assessment, crisis team, hospitalization …).
- Indicate that you would discuss this plan of action with a senior or specialist co-worker.

Alcohol history

Before starting

- Introduce yourself to the patient.
- Establish rapport.
- Explain to the patient that you would like to ask him some questions to evaluate his drinking habits, and ask for his consent to this. As he may be reluctant to give his consent, it is important that you be particularly gentle and tactful.
- Consider using a screening questionnaire such as CAGE (see below).

The CAGE questionnaire

Two 'yes' responses indicate that the possibility of alcoholism should be investigated further. The questionnaire asks the following questions:

1. Have you ever felt you needed to **C**ut down on your drinking?
2. Have people **A**nnoyed you by criticizing your drinking?
3. Have you ever felt **G**uilty about drinking?
4. Have you ever felt you needed a drink first thing in the morning (**E**ye-opener) to steady your nerves or to get rid of a hangover?

The alcohol history

Ask about:

- Alcohol intake:
    - amount
    - type
    - place
    - timing
    - onset and duration
- Features of alcohol dependence:
    1. compulsion to drink/craving
    2. primacy of drinking over other activities
    3. stereotyped pattern of drinking, e.g. narrowing of drinking repertoire
    4. increased tolerance to alcohol, i.e. needing more and more to produce same effect
    5. withdrawal symptoms, e.g. anxiety, sweating, tremor ('the shakes'), nausea, fits, *delirium tremens*. If yes to any of the aforementioned, ask whether withdrawal has been complicated by seizures, or required hospitalization or intensive care unit transfer
    6. relief drinking to avoid withdrawal symptoms, e.g. 'eye opener' first thing in the morning
    7. reinstatement after abstinence

NB. For a diagnosis of alcohol dependence to be made, DSM-IV requires at least three from a similar list of seven features occurring at any time during a 12-month period.

Medical history

Ask about depression and the common medical complications of alcohol abuse, e.g. peptic ulceration, pancreatitis, ischemic heart disease, liver disease, peripheral neuropathy.

Drug history

Note that:

- Illicit drug use is common in alcoholics.
- Alcohol potentiates the effects of certain drugs such as phenytoin.

Family history

Ask about a family history of alcohol or drug abuse.

Social history

Cover employment, housing, marital problems, financial problems, and legal (forensic) problems.

After finishing

- Give the patient feedback on his drinking habits (e.g. amount he drinks versus recommended maximum amount) and, if appropriate, suggest ways for him to cut down his alcohol use.
- Ask him if he has any questions or concerns.
- Thank him for his cooperation.

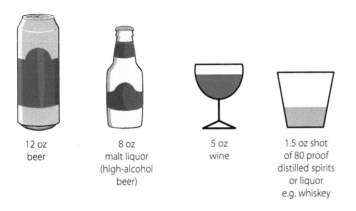

12 oz	8 oz	5 oz	1.5 oz shot
beer	malt liquor	wine	of 80 proof
	(high-alcohol		distilled spirits
	beer)		or liquor
			e.g. whiskey

Figure 39. Equivalences for one standard drink of alcohol. In the USA a standard drink is equal to 14 grams (0.6 oz) of pure alcohol. Note that one bottle of wine is equivalent to approximately 5 standard drinks, and one bottle of spirits (such as rum or vodka) to approximately 17 standard drinks. The Centers for Disease Control and Prevention (CDC) recommend that men should have no more than 2 drinks per day and women should have no more than 1 drink per day when non-pregnant. Total abstinence from alcohol during pregnancy is recommended.

Motivational interviewing

Scenario A

Doctor: According to your blood tests, you appear to be drinking rather too much alcohol.

Patient: I suppose I do enjoy the occasional drink.

Doctor: Are you sure it is just the occasional drink? Alcohol is very bad for you and I think that if you are drinking too much then you really need to stop.

Patient: You sound like my wife.

Doctor: Well, she's right you know. Alcohol can cause liver and heart problems and many other things besides. So you really need to stop drinking, OK?

Patient: Yes, doctor, thank you. (Patient never returns.)

Scenario B (using motivational interviewing)

Doctor: We all enjoy a drink now and then, but sometimes alcohol can do us a lot of harm. What do you know about the harmful effects of alcohol?

Patient: Quite a bit, I'm afraid. My best friend, well he used to drink a lot. Last year he spent three months in hospital. I visited him often, but most of the time he wasn't with it. Then he died from internal bleeding.

Doctor: I'm sorry to hear that, alcohol can really do us a lot of damage.

Patient: It does a lot of damage to the liver, doesn't it?

Doctor: That's right, but it doesn't just do harm to our body, it also does harm to our lives: our work, our finances, our relationships.

Patient: Funny you should say that. My wife's been at my neck…

(…)

Doctor: So, you've told me that you're currently drinking about 9 drinks per day. This has placed severe strain on your marriage and on your relationship with your daughter Emma, not to mention that you haven't been to work since last Tuesday and have started to fear for your job. But what you fear most is ending up lying on a hospital bed like your friend Tom. Is that a fair summary of things as they stand?

Patient: Things are completely out of hand, aren't they? If I don't stop drinking now, I might lose everything I've built over the past 20 years: my job, my marriage, even my daughter.

Doctor: I'm afraid you might be right.

Patient: I really need to quit drinking.

Doctor: You sound very motivated to stop drinking. Why don't we make another appointment to talk about the ways in which we might support you? (…)

This adapted excerpt is from *Psychiatry* 2e, by Neel Burton (Wiley-Blackwell, 2010)

Station 43

Eating disorders history

Before starting

- Introduce yourself to the patient.
- Explain that you are going to ask some questions about his eating habits, and ask for his consent to do this.
- Ensure that he is comfortable.
- If this information is not provided, ask for his name, age, and occupation.

The history

Weight and perception of weight

Determine:

- His current weight and height.
- The amount of weight that he has lost, and over what period.
- Whether the weight loss has been intentional.
- Whether he still considers that he is overweight.
- How often he weighs himself/looks at himself in the mirror.

Diet and compensatory behaviors

Ask about:

- Amount and type of food eaten in an average day.
- Binge eating.
- Vomiting.
- The use of laxatives, purgatives, diuretics, appetite suppressants, and stimulants.
- Physical exercise.

Other

Ask about:

- Menstrual periods.
- Effect on patient's life:
  - relationships
  - medical complications, e.g. anemia, peptic ulceration, constipation
  - psychiatric complications, especially substance misuse, depression, and self harm
- Past medical, drug, and family history (briefly and only if you have time left).

After finishing

- Ask the patient if there is anything he might add that you have forgotten to ask about.
- Determine the patient's level of insight into the problem.
- Thank the patient, offer feedback, and suggest a further course of action, e.g. informant history from the mother, physical examination, investigations, dietary advice, psychotherapy, antidepressants, hospitalization.

Table 18. Anorexia nervosa vs. bulimia nervosa

DSM-IV diagnostic criteria

Anorexia

A. Refusal to maintain normal body weight at more than 85% of expected body weight.

B. Intense fear of gaining weight or becoming fat.

C. Disturbed perception of body weight or shape.

D. In postmenarchal females, amenorrhea for at least three consecutive cycles (if not on the oral contraceptive pill).

Bulimia

A. Recurrent episodes of binge eating.

B. Recurrent inappropriate compensatory behavior to prevent weight gain.

C. Episodes of binge eating and compensatory behavior occur at least twice a week for a period of 3 months.

D. Self-evaluation is unduly influenced by body shape and weight.

E. Disturbance does not occur exclusively during periods of anorexia nervosa.

Capacity and its assessment

In clinical practice or, less commonly, an exam, you may be asked to carry out a formalized assessment of competence to decide on the ability of a patient to give informed consent (see *Station 86*). Alternatively, you may simply be asked to discuss the subject.

The first thing to note is that the terms capacity and competence are often used interchangeably but, strictly speaking, capacity is the legal presumption that adult persons have the ability to make decisions, whereas competence is a clinical determination of a patient's ability to make decisions about his treatment.

Consent capacity is central to the medical–legal doctrine of informed consent, which requires that a valid consent to treatment be informed, voluntary, and competent. In Section 1(3), the Uniform Health-Care Decisions Act ('B71' National Conference of Commissioners on Uniform State Laws, 1993) defines consent capacity as 'the ability to understand significant benefits, risks, and alternatives to proposed health care and to make and communicate a health-care decision'. See Moye, J. & Marson, D. C. (2009) Assessment of decision-making capacity in older adults: an emerging area of practice and research. *Focus*, **7**: 88–97.

Issues about capacity frequently arise in three groups of patients: children and adolescents, patients with learning difficulties, and patients with mental illness. A person has capacity so long as he has the ability to understand and retain relevant information for long enough to reach a *reasoned* decision, **regardless of the actual decision reached**. An adult person should be presumed to have the competence to make a particular decision until a judgement about capacity can be made. This judgement can only be made about present capacity, not about past or future capacity, and it should only be made for a specific decision, as different decisions require different levels of capacity. The doctor in charge has the responsibility to act in the best interests of the patient. Nevertheless, it is good practice for him to involve co-workers, caregivers, and relatives in the decision-making. In difficult situations, or if there are differences of opinion about the patient's best interests, the doctor should consult a senior co-worker or seek legal advice.

Assessing capacity

1. Ensure that the patient understands:
    - what the intervention is
    - why the intervention is being proposed
    - the alternatives to the intervention, including no intervention
    - the principal benefits and risks of the intervention and of its alternatives
    - the consequences of the intervention and of its alternatives
2. Ensure that the patient retains the information for long enough to weigh it in the balance and reach a reasoned decision, whatever that decision might be. In some cases, the patient may not have the cognitive ability or emotional maturity to reach a reasoned decision, or may be unduly affected by mental illness.
3. Ensure that the patient is not subject to coercion or threat.

It is important to bear in mind that a patient's capacity can be enhanced by, for example:

- making your explanations easier to understand, e.g. using diagrams
- seeing the patient at his best time of day
- seeing the patient with a friend or relative
- improving the patient's environment, e.g. finding a quiet side-room
- adjusting the patient's medication, e.g. decreasing the dose of sedative drugs

Hearing and the ear examination

Before starting

- Introduce yourself to the patient.
- Explain the examination and ask for his consent to carry it out.
- Sit him so that he is facing you and ensure that he is comfortable.

The history

- Name, age, and occupation, if this information has not already been provided.
- Ask the patient if there has been any loss of hearing.

If there has been loss of hearing, assess its:

- Characteristics (bilaterality, onset, duration, severity, impact on the patient's life).
- Associated features (tinnitus, vertigo, pain, discharge, weight loss).
- Possible causes (noise exposure, trauma, infection, antibiotics, family history).
- Impact on the patient's life.
- Previous ear problems.

The examination

Hearing

Test hearing by rubbing your fingers together softly, whilst distracting or occluding the other ear.

Tuning fork tests

 Use a 512 Hz tuning fork, and not the larger 128 Hz or 256 Hz tuning forks used for neurological examinations.

- The Rinne test. Place the base of the vibrating tuning fork on the mastoid process of each ear. Once the patient can no longer 'hear' the vibration, move the tuning fork in front of the ear. If the tuning fork can be heard, air conduction is better than bone conduction, and there is therefore no conductive hearing loss. The test is said to be *positive*. If the tuning fork cannot be heard, there is a conductive hearing loss, and the test is said to be *negative*.

 The false negative Rinne test: if the Rinne test is performed on a deaf ear, it may appear negative because the vibration is transmitted to the opposite ear.

- The Weber test. Place the vibrating tuning fork in the midline of the skull. If hearing is normal, or if hearing loss is symmetrical, the vibration should be heard equally in both ears.

Note:

- If there is conductive deafness in one ear, the vibration is best heard *in that same ear* (since there is no background interference).
- If there is sensorineural deafness in one ear, the vibration is best heard in the other ear.

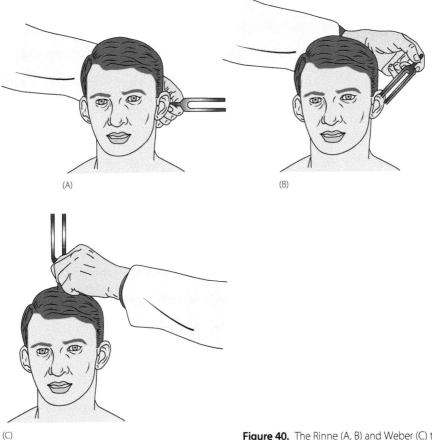

(A)

(B)

(C)

Figure 40. The Rinne (A, B) and Weber (C) tests.

Otoscopy

- Examine the pinnae for size, shape, deformities, pre-auricular sinuses.
- Look behind the ears for any scars.
- Palpate the pre-auricular, post-auricular, and infra-auricular lymph nodes.
- Affix a speculum of appropriate size onto the otoscope.
- Gently pull the pinna upward and backward so as to straighten the ear canal and, holding the otoscope like a pen (see *Figure 41*), introduce it into the external auditory meatus.

 If examining the right ear, use your right hand to hold the otoscope. If examining the left ear, use your left hand.

- Through the otoscope, inspect the ear canal (discharge, foreign body, wax, exotosis, otitis externa) and the tympanic membrane (normal anatomy, color (normally pearly gray), shape (normally concave), light reflex (normally present), effusions, cholesteatomata, perforations, grommets).

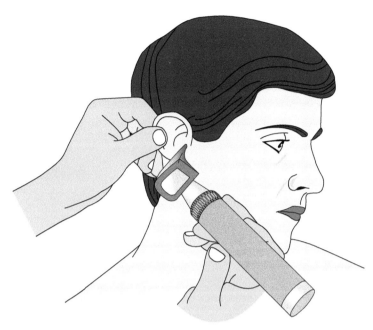

Figure 41. Holding the otoscope.

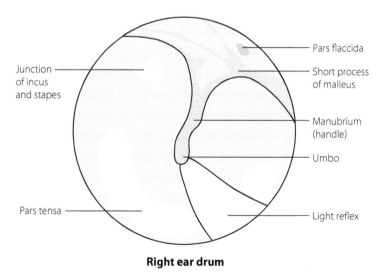

Junction
of incus
and stapes

Pars flaccida

Short process
of malleus

Manubrium
(handle)

Umbo

Pars tensa

Light reflex

Right ear drum

Figure 42. The normal right ear drum.

After examining the ear

- Ask the patient if he has any questions or concerns.
- Thank the patient.
- Summarize your findings and offer a differential diagnosis, e.g. ear wax, otitis media, perforated ear drum.

Clinical Skills for Medical Students

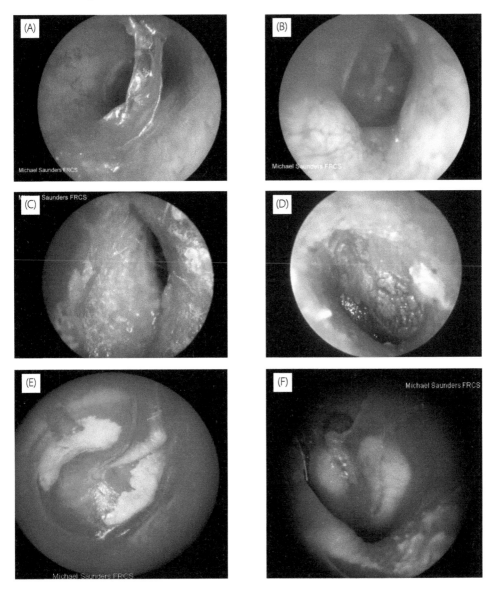

Figure 43. Common ear problems.

(A) Wax: excess or impacted wax, can occlude the ear canal.

(B) Exostoses: bony swellings in the ear canal due to chronic cold water exposure, can cause pain and predispose to infection or occlusion of the ear canal.

(C) Otitis externa: inflammation of the outer ear and ear canal, associated with pain, can cause swelling and discharge and occlusion of the ear canal – pain is typically exacerbated by pulling on the pinna or pushing on the tragus.

(D) Acute otitis media: inflammation of the middle ear due to infection, associated with pain, redness and bulging of the tympanic membrane, disintegration of the light reflex, effusions, perforation.

(E) Tympanosclerosis: calcium deposits in the ear drum due to trauma or infection, can lead to impairment of hearing.

(F) Cholesteatoma: destructive growth of keratinizing squamous epithelium in the middle ear, often due to a tear or retraction of the ear drum, can lead to impairment of hearing.

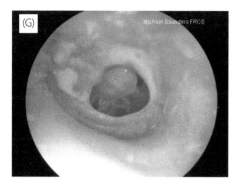

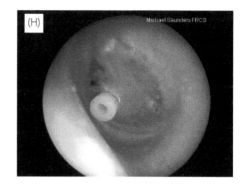

Figure 43. Common ear problems – *continued*.

(G) Perforation.
(H) Grommet: small tube inserted in chronic otitis media to drain and ventilate the middle ear.

Reproduced with permission from Michael Saunders, Bristol Royal Infirmary, UK

Conditions most likely to come up in a hearing and the ear examination
Conductive hearing loss:
• commonly caused by wax, foreign bodies, exostoses, otitis externa, otitis media, trauma or damage to the ear drum or ossicles
Sensorineural hearing loss:
• may be caused by noise exposure, degenerative changes (presbyacusis), trauma, infection, aminoglycoside drugs such as gentamicin, Ménière's disease, acoustic neuroma

Station 46

Vision and the eye examination (including fundoscopy)

Before starting

- Introduce yourself to the patient.
- Explain the examination and ask for his consent to carry it out.
- Ensure that he is comfortable.

The examination

1. Visual acuity

- *Snellen chart.* Assess each eye individually, either from a distance of 6 m or 3 m (20 feet or 10 feet, respectively), correcting for any refractive errors (glasses, pinhole). If the patient cannot read the Snellen chart, either move him closer or ask him to count fingers. If he fails to count fingers, test whether he can see hand movements and, if he cannot, test whether he can see light.
- *Test types* (or fine print). Assess each eye individually, correcting for any refractive errors.
- *Ishihara plates.* Indicate that you could use Ishihara plates to test color vision specifically.

2. Visual fields

- *Confrontation test.* Test the visual fields by confrontation. Sit directly opposite the patient, at the same level as him. Ask him to look straight at you and to cover his right eye with his right hand. Cover your left eye with your left hand, and test the visual field of his left eye with your right hand. Bring a wiggly finger into the upper left quadrant, asking the patient to say when he sees the finger. Repeat for the lower left quadrant. Then swap hands and test the upper and lower right quadrants. Now ask the patient to cover his left eye with his left hand. Cover your right eye with your right hand and test the visual field of his right eye with your left hand. Bring a wiggly finger into the upper right quadrant, asking the patient to say when he sees the finger. Repeat for the lower right quadrant. Then swap hands and test the upper and lower left quadrants.
- *Mapping of central visual field defects.* Indicate that you could use a red pin to delineate the patient's blind spot and any central visual field defects.
- *Visual inattention test.* Ask the patient to fix his gaze upon you and simultaneously bring a moving finger into each of the patient's right and left visual fields. In some parietal lobe lesions, only the ipsilateral finger is perceived by the patient.

3. Pupillary reflexes

- *Inspection.* Inspect the eyes, paying particular attention to the size and symmetry of the pupils, and excluding a visible ptosis or squint.
- Test the direct and consensual pupillary light reflexes. Explain that you are going to shine a bright light into the patient's eye and that this may feel uncomfortable. Bring the light in onto his left eye and look for pupil constriction. Bring the light in onto his left eye once again, but this time look for pupil constriction in his *right eye* (consensual reflex). Repeat for the right eye.
- Perform the swinging flashlight test. Swing the light from one eye to another and look for sustained pupil constriction in both eyes. Intermittent pupil constriction in one eye (Marcus Gunn pupil) suggests a lesion of the optic nerve anterior to the optic chiasm.
- Test the accommodation reflex. Ask the patient to follow your finger in to his nose. As the eyes converge, the pupils should constrict.

4. Eye movements

- Perform the cover test. Ask the patient to fixate on a point and cover one eye. Observe the movement of the uncovered eye. Repeat the test for the other eye.
- Examine eye movements. Ask the patient to keep his head still and to follow your finger with his eyes. Ask him to report any pain or double vision at any point. Draw an 'H' shape with your finger.
- *Nystagmus*. Look out for nystagmus at the extremes of gaze. You can do this as part of eye movements or separately by fixing the patient's head and asking him to track your finger through a cross pattern.

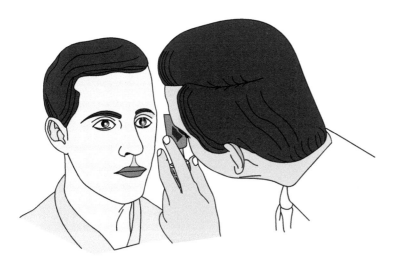

Figure 44. Holding the ophthalmoscope.

5. Fundoscopy

Explain the procedure, mentioning that it may be uncomfortable. Darken the room and ask the patient to fixate on a distant object (or to 'look over my shoulder'). In an exam, state that, ideally, the pupils should have been dilated using a solution of 1% tropicamide.

- *Red reflex.* Test the red reflex in each eye from a distance of about 10 cm. An absent red reflex is usually caused by a cataract, but in children consider a retinoblastoma.
- *Fundoscopy.* Use your right eye to examine the patient's right eye, and your left eye to examine the patient's left eye. If you use your left eye to examine the patient's right eye, you may appear more caring than the examiner might like to see. Look at the optic disc, the blood vessels, and the macula. To find the macula, ask the patient to look directly into the light. Describe any features according to protocol, e.g. *"There are soft exudates at 3 o'clock, two disc diameters away from the disc".*

 If the station is examining fundoscopy alone, the patient is likely to be replaced by a model in which the retinas are very easy to visualize. Before the exam, it is a good idea to look at as many retinas as you can, both in patients and in textbooks/on the internet.

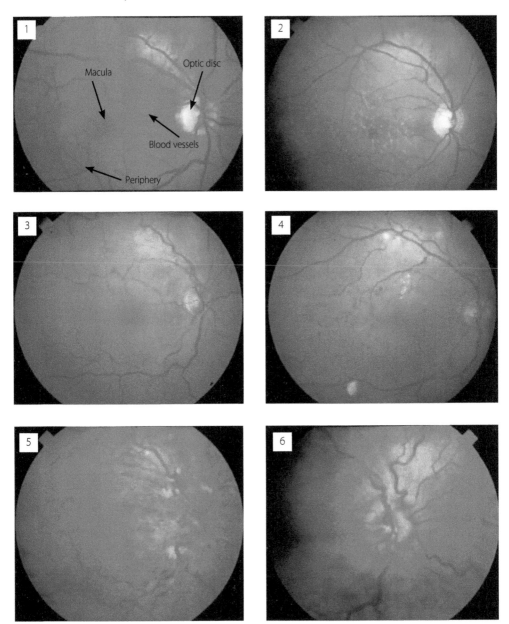

Figure 45. Findings on fundoscopy of the right eye.
1. Normal.
2. Senile macular degeneration.
3. Hypertensive retinopathy.
4. Pre-proliferative diabetic retinopathy.
5. Central retinal vein occlusion.
6. Papilledema.

After the examination

- Ask the patient if he has any questions or concerns.
- Thank the patient.
- Summarize your findings and offer a differential diagnosis.

Conditions most likely to come up in a vision and the eye examination

Cataract:
- absent red reflex, on approaching ophthalmoscope the lens may look like cracked ice

Senile macular degeneration:
- drusen (characteristic yellow deposits) in the macula, exudative changes resulting from blood and fluid under the macula

Hypertensive retinopathy:
- stage I: arteriolar narrowing and tortuosity
- stage II: AV nicking, silver-wiring
- stage III: dot, blot, and flame hemorrhages, microaneurysms, soft exudates ('cotton wool spots'), hard exudates
- stage IV: papilledema

Diabetic retinopathy:
- background: microaneurysms, macular edema, hard exudates, hemorrhages
- pre-proliferative: 'cotton wool spots', venous beading
- proliferative: neovascularization, vitreous hemorrhage

Glaucoma:
- increased cup to disk ratio (> 0.5), hemorrhages

Central retinal artery occlusion:
- pale retina with swelling or edema, markedly decreased vascularity, cherry red spot in the central fovea

Central retinal vein occlusion:
- widespread hemorrhages throughout the retina with swelling and edema, sometimes described as a 'stormy sunset'

Papilledema:
- blurring of disc margins, cupping and swelling of the disc, hemorrhages, exudates, distended veins

Smell and the nose examination

Specifications: This station may involve a model of a nose in lieu of a patient.

Before starting

- Introduce yourself to the patient.
- Explain the examination and ask him for his consent to carry it out.
- Position him so that he is sitting in a chair facing you.
- Ensure that he is comfortable.

The history

- Briefly establish the nature of the problem.
- If there is obstruction of the nasal passages, determine its:
  - characteristics (nasal passage affected, onset, duration, timing, severity)
  - associated symptoms (facial pain, inflammation, itching, rhinorrhea, sneezing, snoring, anosmia)
  - possible causes (asthma, hay fever, other allergies, trauma, surgery, other)
  - impact on everyday life

The examination

Inspection

- Observe the external appearance of the nose from the front, from the side, and from above. Look for evidence of deformity, inflammation, nasal discharge, skin disease, and scars.
- Examine the nasal vestibule, anterior end of the septum, and anterior ends of the inferior turbinates. Do this first by elevating the tip of the nose, and then with the help of a Thudicum speculum and flashlight.
- Look into the mouth.

Otoscopy

- Use an otoscope in conjunction with a Thudicum speculum to assess the nasal septum and the inferior and middle turbinates. Make sure that the otoscope has a very wide end-piece on it. Look for septal deviation, mucosal inflammation, bleeding, perforation, polyps, and foreign objects.

 A more detailed view of the nasal cavities can be obtained using a flexible (fiber-optic) nasendoscope.

Nasal airflow

- Ask the patient to breathe out through his nose onto a mirror or cold tongue depressor positioned under the nose. If the nasal passages are not obstructed, there should be condensation under both nostrils.
- Assess inspiratory flow by occluding one nostril and asking the patient to sniff. Repeat for the other side.

ENT, ophthalmology, and dermatology

Smell

- Assess sense of smell by asking the patient to identify fragrances from a series of bottles containing different odors.

Sinuses

- With your thumb, press over the supra- and infra-orbital areas to elicit tenderness. Tenderness in these areas is likely to indicate inflammation of the frontal and maxillary sinuses (sinusitis).

After examining the nose

- Ask the patient if he has any questions or concerns.
- Thank the patient.
- In an exam, offer to examine the throat and ears.
- Summarize your findings and offer a differential diagnosis.

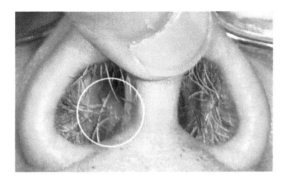

Figure 46. Nasal polyp. Swollen turbinates are often mistaken for polyps. However, swollen turbinates differ from polyps in that they tend to be pink rather than gray/yellow in colour, and in that they tend to be sensitive rather than insensitive to touch.

Reproduced from www.askdrshah.com with permission from Dr Rajesh Shah.

Conditions most likely to come up in a smell and nose examination station
• Congenital or trauma-induced deviated nasal septum
• Septum perforation secondary to cocaine use, nose picking, or granulomatous disease
• Chronic rhinitis
• Nasal polyps
• Anosmia secondary to viral infection or head injury

Station 48

Lump in the neck examination

Before starting

- Introduce yourself to the patient.
- Explain the examination and ask for his consent to carry it out.
- Ask him to expose his neck and upper body.
- Sit him in a chair.

The examination

Inspection

- Inspect the patient generally, in particular looking for any signs of thyroid disease. The age and sex of the patient has an important bearing on the differential diagnosis of a goiter.
- Inspect the neck from the front and side, looking for goiter, other lumps, scars, and any other abnormalities.

 A goiter, or enlarged thyroid gland, is seen as a swelling below the cricoid cartilage, on either side of the trachea.

- Ask the patient to take a sip of water. The following structures move upon swallowing: thyroid gland, thyroid cartilage, cricoid cartilage, thyroglossal cyst, lymph nodes.
- Ask him to stick his tongue out. A midline swelling which moves upward when the tongue is protruded is a thyroglossal cyst.

Palpation

- Ask him if there is any tenderness in the neck area.
- Putting one hand on either side of his neck, examine the anterior and posterior triangles of the neck with your fingertips. For any lump, assess its site, size, shape, surface, consistency, and fixity. Is the lump tender to touch? Note that the normal thyroid gland is often not palpable.
- Palpate the cervical lymph nodes.
- Palpate for tracheal deviation in the suprasternal notch (see *Station 22: Respiratory system examination*).

Percussion

- Percuss for the dullness of a retrosternal goiter over the sternum and upper chest.

Auscultation

- Auscultate over the thyroid for bruits. Ask the patient to hold his breath as you listen; a soft bruit is sometimes heard in thyrotoxicosis.

Assessment of thyroid function

- Examine the patient for signs of hyper- and hypothyroidism, as appropriate (see below). Once you have examined the neck, this involves examining the hands (temperature, nails, skin, hair, tremor, pulse) and the eyes (chemosis, lid retraction, lid lag, periorbital edema, proptosis, ophthalmoplegia and diplopia), and looking for evidence of congestive cardiac failure, pre-tibial myxedema, and hyporeflexia. To look for exophthalmos, stand behind the patient and look at the eyes from above. To look for lid lag and ophthalmoplegia, test eye movements and ask the patient to tell you if he sees double at any time. If asked, you can offer to objectively measure the degree of proptosis using an exophthalmometer.

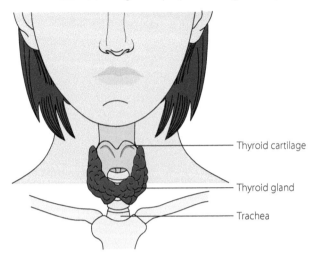

Thyroid cartilage

Thyroid gland

Trachea

Figure 47. Anatomy of the normal thyroid gland.

After the examination

- Help the patient to put his clothes back on.
- Ensure that he is comfortable.
- Ask him if he has any questions or concerns.
- Thank him.
- Offer a diagnosis or differential diagnosis.
- Give suggestions for further management, e.g. thyroid function tests, thyroid antibodies, ultrasound examination of the thyroid, iodine thyroid scan, fine needle aspiration cytology.

Goiters and thyroid disease

Signs of **hyperthyroidism**: enlarged thyroid gland or thyroid nodules, thyroid bruit, hyperthermia, diaphoresis, dehydration, tremor, tachycardia, arrhythmia, congestive cardiac failure, onycholysis.

- Graves' disease (commonest cause of hyperthyroidism): uniformly enlarged smooth thyroid gland usually in a younger patient; lid retraction, lid lag, chemosis, periorbital edema, proptosis, diplopia, pre-tibial myxedema (non-pitting edema and skin thickening, seen in <5% of cases), thyroid acropachy (finger clubbing, seen in <1% of cases).
- Toxic multinodular goiter: enlarged multinodular goiter in a middle-aged patient.
- Toxic nodule and de Quervain's thyroiditis are less common.

Signs of **hypothyroidism**: hypothermia and cold intolerance, weight gain, slowed speech and movements, hoarse voice, dry skin, hair loss, coarse facial features and facial puffiness, hypotension, bradycardia, and hyporeflexia.

- Hashimoto's thyroiditis (commonest cause of hypothyroidism): moderately enlarged rubbery thyroid gland, usually in a female patient aged 30–50 years; initial hyperthyroidism that progresses to hypothyroidism and, if untreated, to myxedema.

[Note]   Iodine deficiency can also cause a goiter but this is rarely seen in developed countries.

Clinical Skills for Medical Students

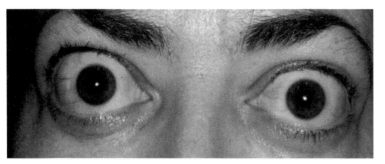

Figure 48. Eye signs in Graves' disease.
Reproduced from www.eyeplastics.net.

Conditions most likely to appear in a lump in the neck examination station
Toxic goiter:
• diffuse (Graves' disease), multinodular, toxic nodule (see above)
Hashimoto's thyroiditis (see above)
Physiological goiter of puberty or pregnancy (or both)
Thyroglossal cyst:
• fibrous cyst that forms from a persistent thyroglossal duct
• midline lump in the region of the hyoid bone that is smooth and cystic and usually painless
• moves upward upon swallowing and upon tongue protrusion
Enlarged lymph nodes
NB. Other, less likely, possibilities include thyroid carcinoma, branchial cyst, cystic hygroma (lymphangioma), carotid body tumor, and sternocleidomastoid tumor.

Dermatological history

Before starting

- Introduce yourself to the patient.
- Explain that you are going to ask him some questions to uncover the nature of his skin problem, and ask for his consent to do this.
- Ensure that he is comfortable; if not, make sure that he is.

The history

- Name and age.

Chief complaint

- Use an open question to ask the patient to describe his skin problem.

History of presenting illness

Ask about:

- When, where, and how the problem started.
- What the initial lesions looked like and how they have evolved. Are the hair and nails also involved?
- Symptoms: especially, pain, pruritus, blistering and bleeding.
- Aggravating factors such as sunlight, heat, soaps, etc.
- Relieving factors, including any treatments so far.
- Effect on everyday life.
- Details of previous episodes, if any.

Past medical history

- Previous skin disease.
- Atopy (asthma, allergic rhinitis, childhood eczema).
- Present and past medical illnesses.
- Surgery.

Drug history

- Prescribed and OTC/complementary medications, including topical applications such as gels and creams.
- Cosmetics and moisturizing creams.
- Relationship of symptoms to use of medication.
- Allergies.

Family history

- Has anyone in the family had a similar problem?
- Medical history of parents, siblings, and children, focusing on skin problems.
- Sexual contacts.

Social history

- Occupation (in some detail). Has the patient's occupation exposed him to any allergens or irritants? Have co-workers been suffering from similar symptoms? Do the symptoms improve during time off work?
- Hobbies (in some detail). Have the patient's hobbies exposed him to any allergens or irritants? Has he been using sunbeds?
- Home circumstances.
- Alcohol use.
- Smoking.
- Recent travel, especially to the tropics.

Systems review

(If appropriate.)

After taking the history

- Ask the patient if there is anything that he might add that you have forgotten to ask about.
- Thank the patient.
- Summarize your findings and offer a differential diagnosis.
- In an exam, state that you should next like to carry out a dermatological examination.

Dermatological examination

Before starting

- Introduce yourself to the patient.
- Explain the examination and ask for his consent to carry it out.
- Ask him to undress to his undergarments.
- Ensure that he is comfortable.
- Ask him to report any pain or discomfort during the examination.
- Ensure that there is adequate lighting.

The examination

- Describe the distribution of the lesions: are they generalized or localized, symmetrical or asymmetrical, affecting only certain areas, e.g. flexor or extensor surfaces. Make a point of looking at all parts of the body.
- Describe the morphology of the individual lesions, commenting upon their color, size, shape, borders, elevation, and spatial relationship. Use precise dermatological terms. A glossary of dermatological terms with accompanying images can be found at: www.dermnetnz.org/terminology.html.
- Note any secondary skin lesions such as scaling, lichenification, crusting, excoriation, erosion, ulceration, and scarring.
- Palpate the lesions (ask the patient if this is OK first). Assess their consistency. Do they blanch?
- Examine the finger nails and toe nails.
- Examine the hair and scalp.
- Examine the mucous membranes.
- Check for lymphadenopathy, if appropriate.
- Check the pedal pulses, if appropriate.

After the examination

- If appropriate, offer to help the patient to put his clothes back on.
- Thank the patient.
- Ensure that he is comfortable.
- Wash your hands.
- Summarize your findings and offer a differential diagnosis.

Senior Resident's questions

Differentiating skin cancers

BCC (75% of skin cancers) most often looks like a pearly bump or nodule on sun-exposed areas of skin. Bleeding or crusting may develop in the center of the tumor, as in the photograph below. In contrast, squamous cell carcinoma (SCC, 20% of all skin cancers) most often looks a red, scaling, thickened patch, sometimes with bleeding, crusting, or ulceration. Although less common than either BCC or SCC, malignant melanoma is more commonly fatal. Pigmented lesions of the skin should be suspected to be malignant melanomas if they are **a**symmetrical, if they have irregular **b**orders, if their **c**olor varies from one area to another, or if their **d**iameter is larger than that of a pencil eraser (6 mm). This is easily remembered as A, B, C, D.

(A)

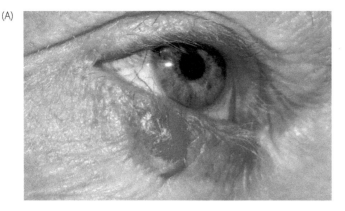

(B)

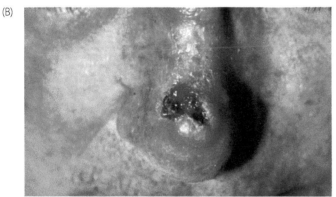

Figure 49. (A) Basal cell carcinoma (BCC). Reproduced from http://picasaweb.google.com/schalock. (B) Squamous cell carcinoma. Reproduced from http://commons.wikimedia.org/wiki/filesquamous_cell_carcinoma.jpg

---

Conditions most likely to come up in a skin examination station

Psoriasis:

- chronic, autoimmune skin disease
- plaque psoriasis is most common type (c. 90%)
- red plaques with silvery scales due to inflammation and excessive skin production
- frequently on the elbows or knees, but can also affect any area including the scalp, palms, and soles
- may be accompanied by nail dystrophy
- may be accompanied by joint inflammation (psoriatic arthritis)
- may be aggravated by stress, alcohol, smoking, and certain drugs, e.g. lithium, beta blockers, chloroquinine

Eczema:

- most common types are atopic or flexural eczema and irritant-induced contact dermatitis
- recurrent dryness, itching, and skin rashes that may be accompanied by redness, inflammation, cracking, weeping, blistering, crusting, flaking, and skin discoloration
- frequently on the flexor aspects of joints (cf. psoriasis)

Acne vulgaris:

- changes in the pilosebaceous units as a result of increased androgen stimulation
- comedones (blackheads), inflammatory papules, pustules, and nodules that affect the face and neck and also the chest, back, and shoulders, and that can result in scarring
- usually appears during adolescence and may persist into early adulthood

Rosacea:

- chronic condition that primarily affects fair-skinned people and that is 2–3 times more common in women
- peak age of onset is 30–50
- typically begins as flushing and redness on the central face
- may be accompanied by telangiectasia, red domed papules and pustules, red gritty eyes, burning and stinging sensations, and, in some advanced cases, a red lobulated nose (rhinophyma)
- may be aggravated by stress, sunlight, cold weather, alcohol

Skin cancer (see *Senior Resident's questions* above)

Station 51

Clinical Skills for Medical Students

Advice on sun protection

 Read in conjunction with Station 85: Explaining skills.

Before starting

- Introduce yourself to the patient.
- Tell him what you are going to explain, and determine how much he already knows.

The advice

Explain that there are three types of ultraviolet radiation from the sun: UVA, UVB, and UVC.

- UVA and UVB can cause skin cancer.
- UVC does not reach the surface of the earth and is therefore of no concern.

Explain that, other than causing skin cancer, UV radiation can also cause the skin to burn and (horror!) to age prematurely.

UV levels depend on a number of factors such as the time of day, time of year, latitude, altitude, cloud cover, and ozone cover.

Explain that there are four principal methods of protecting against the sun's rays:

1. Avoid the outdoors. The sun's rays are most direct around midday and so one should avoid being outdoors from around 11 am to 3 pm.
2. Seek shade.
3. Cover up (clothing should include a wide-brimmed hat and sunglasses that conform to US Standard ANSI Z80.3-2001, British and European Standard 1836:2005, or Australian Standard AS/NZS 1067:2003).
4. Use sunscreen.
   - A sunscreen's star rating is a measure of its level of protection against UVA.
   - A sunscreen's sun protection factor is a measure of its level of protection against UVB.
   - Use a sunscreen that has a star rating of at least three stars *** and an SPF of at least 15.
   - The sunscreen should be applied thickly over all sun-exposed areas, and re-applied regularly.

 It is important that you explain that sunscreens should not simply be used as a means of spending more time in the sun.

Finally advise the patient to report any moles that change in size, shape, color, or texture.

After giving the advice

- Summarize the information and ensure that the patient has understood it.
- Tell them that, if anything, they can remember 'Slip, slap, slop' – slip on some clothes, slap on a hat, and slop on sunscreen.
- Ask the patient if he has any questions or concerns.
- Give the patient a leaflet on sun protection.

Examination of a superficial mass and of lymph nodes

Before starting

- Introduce yourself to the patient.
- If allowed, take a brief history from him, for example, onset, course, effect on everyday life.
- Explain the examination and ask for his consent.
- Ask him to expose the lump completely.
- Position him appropriately and ensure that he is comfortable.

The examination

- Inspect the patient from the end of the bed, looking for other lumps and any other signs.
- Inspect the lump and note its site, color, and any changes to the overlying skin such as inflammation or tethering. Note also the presence or absence of a punctum.
- Ask the patient if the lump is painful before you palpate it. Is the pain only brought on by palpation or is it a more constant pain?
- Warm your hands.
- Assess the temperature of the lump with the back of your hand.
- Palpate the lump in a rotary motion with the pads of your fingers. Now consider:
  - number: solitary or multiple
  - size: estimate length, width, and height, or use a ruler or measuring tape
  - shape: spherical, ovoid, irregular, other
  - edge: well or poorly defined
  - surface: smooth or irregular
  - consistency: soft, firm, hard, rubbery
  - fluctuance: rest two fingers of your left hand on either side of the lump and press on the lump with the index finger of your right hand: if your left hand fingers are displaced, the lump is fluctuant
  - pulsatility: rest a finger of each hand on either side of the lump: if your fingers are displaced, the lump is pulsatile
  - mobility or fixation both of the overlying skin to the lump, and of the lump to the underlying muscle
  - compressibility and reducibility: press firmly on the lump to see if it disappears; if it immediately reappears, it is compressible; if it only reappears upon standing or coughing, it is reducible
- Percuss the lump for dullness or resonance.
- Auscultate the lump for bruits or bowel sounds.
- Transilluminate the lump by holding it between the fingers of one hand and shining a pen flashlight to it with the other. A bright red glow indicates fluid whereas a dull or absent glow suggests a solid mass.
- Examine the draining lymph nodes (see further down), or indicate that you would do so.

After examining the lump

- Ask the patient if he has any questions or concerns.
- Thank the patient.
- Summarize your findings and offer a differential diagnosis.
- If appropriate, suggest further investigations, e.g. aspirate, biopsy, ultrasound, CT.

Lymph node examination

Head and neck

The patient should be sitting up and examined from behind. With the fingers of both hands, palpate the submental, submandibular, parotid, and pre- and post-auricular nodes. Next palpate the anterior and posterior cervical nodes and the occipital nodes.

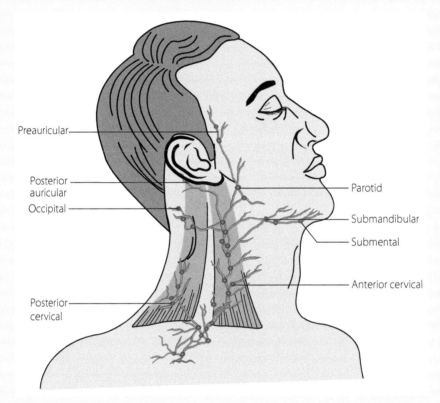

Preauricular

Posterior auricular

Occipital

Posterior cervical

Parotid

Submandibular

Submental

Anterior cervical

Figure 50. Lymph nodes in the head and neck.

Upper body
- Palpate the supraclavicular and infraclavicular nodes on either side of the clavicle.
- Expose the right axilla by lifting and abducting the arm and supporting it at the wrist with your right hand.
- With your left hand, palpate the following lymph node groups:
  - the apical
  - the anterior
  - the posterior
  - the nodes of the medial aspect of the humerus
- Now expose the left axilla by lifting and abducting the left arm and supporting at the wrist with your left hand.
- With your right hand, palpate the lymph node groups, as listed above.

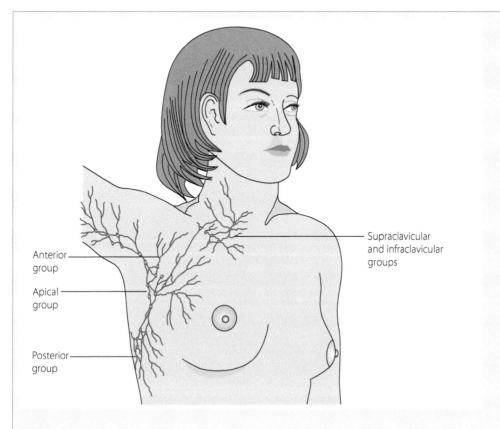

Anterior group

Apical group

Posterior group

Supraclavicular and infraclavicular groups

Figure 51. Lymph nodes of the upper body.

Lower body

Palpate the superficial inguinal nodes (horizontal and vertical), which lie below the inguinal ligament and near the great saphenous vein respectively, then the popliteal node in the popliteal fossa.

Common causes of an isolated superficial lump	
Epidermoid (sebaceous) cyst: • results from obstruction of sebaceous gland • may be red, hot, and tender • spherical, smooth • attached to the skin but not to the underlying muscle • may have a punctum which may exude a cottage cheese discharge	**Fibroma:** • common and benign fibrous tissue tumor • skin-colored and painless • can be sessile or pedunculated, 'hard' or 'soft' • situated in the skin and so unattached to underlying structures
Lipoma: • common and benign soft tissue tumor • skin-colored and painless • spherical, soft and sometimes fluctuant • not attached to the skin and therefore mobile and 'slippery'	**Skin abscess:** • collection of pus in the skin • very likely to be red, hot, and tender • may be indurated

Pediatric history

General points:

- As a rule of thumb, the older the child the more he should be involved in the history-taking process.
- Observe the child's behavior as you take the history.
- The parent's concerns and the child's concerns are likely to differ: try as much as possible to address both.

Before starting

- Introduce yourself to the parent and child (in that order).
- Explain that you are going to ask some questions and obtain consent to do this.
- Ensure that the patient is comfortable; younger children may need some toys to keep them distracted.

The history

- Ask the age, sex, and preferred name of the child.
- Confirm the relationship of the accompanying adult.

Chief complaint and history of presenting illness

- Ask about the nature of the chief complaint and how it has affected the child's daily routine. Start by using open questions and then explore the symptoms as you might in any other history. Ask about onset, duration, previous episodes, pain, associated symptoms (e.g. nausea, vomiting, diarrhea, urinary frequency, constipation, altered consciousness), and treatments.

 Do not under any circumstances denigrate, or omit to address, the parent's concerns.

Systems review

- The major systems should be covered briefly, placing the emphasis on areas of particular relevance.
  - *General health*: liveliness, change in behavior, feeding, fever.
  - *ENT*: sore throat, earache, infections, deafness, nose bleeds.
  - *CVS and RS*: breathing problems (feeding problems in young infants), shortness of breath, exercise tolerance, color changes (blue attacks, pallor), cough, croup, wheeze, stridor, chest infections, heart murmurs.
  - *GIS*: weight gain, feeding, vomiting, diarrhea, constipation, jaundice, abdominal pain.
  - *GUS*: frequency, discharge, enuresis.
  - *NS*: headaches, fits, visual disturbances, balance and co-ordination, muscle problems.
  - *MSS*: limps, joint stiffness, pain, swelling, redness.
  - *Skin*: rash, eczema.

Past medical history

Similar problems in the past?

Ask about these topics if you think that they might be relevant to the child's chief complaint.

- Medical problems (epilepsy, diabetes, asthma, etc.)

- Surgery.
- Birth history:
  - maternal obstetric history (illnesses or infections during pregnancy, blood pressure, fetal growth, drugs during pregnancy, e.g. anti-convulsants, narcotics, smoking, alcohol)
  - mode of delivery and any problems
  - gestation at delivery
  - birth weight
  - problems after birth and admission to Neonatal Intensive Care Unit
- Developmental milestones (smiling, sitting, walking and talking – see *Station 54: Developmental assessment*).
- Feeding (breast, bottle, how long, how much).
- Sleeping patterns.
- Childhood illnesses.
- Immunizations.

Drug history

- Prescribed and over-the-counter medications.
- Allergies.

Family history

- Health of parents and siblings.
- Congenital/genetic abnormalities. (*"Are there any illnesses that run in the family?"*)
- Cosanguinity.

Social history

- Parental occupation.
- Details of home life, siblings.
- Behavior at home and at school.
- Pets and smokers in the home (if relevant).

After taking the history

- Ask the parent if there is anything that he/she might add that you have forgotten to ask about.
- Ask the parent and child if they have any specific questions or concerns.
- Thank the parent and child.
- Summarize your findings and offer a differential diagnosis.

Conditions most likely to come up in a pediatric history station

- Respiratory conditions, e.g. asthma, upper respiratory tract infection
- Headache
- Behavioral problems, e.g. enuresis
- Fits, e.g. febrile convulsions, epilepsy
- Childhood infections/rashes and immunization compliance.

Developmental assessment

Development in the early years of life is fairly consistent from child to child and any significant deviation from this pattern is thus a reliable marker of pathology.

The four parameters by which development is assessed

1. Gross motor skills
2. Vision and fine movement
3. Hearing and language
4. Social behavior

Key ages for developmental assessment

1. Newborn
2. Supine infant (1.5–2 months)
3. Sitting infant (6–9 months)
4. Toddler (18–24 months)
5. Communicating child (3–4 years)

The developmental assessment

Specifications: This station may require you to carry out a developmental assessment or watch a short video and answer some questions about it.

The developmental assessment is usually performed alongside a general history, so many of the subject headings are the same as in *Station 53: Pediatric history*. Remember to tailor the assessment to the age of the child and that much of the assessment can and should be carried out by observation alone.

Before starting

- Introduce yourself to the parent and child.
- Explain that you are going to ask some questions and obtain consent to do this.
- Ensure that the child is comfortable; younger children may need toys to keep them distracted.
- Ask for the child's developmental log, if one is available.

The assessment

- Ask for the age, sex, and preferred name of the child.

Chief complaint and history of presenting illness

- Ask about the nature of the chief complaint and its effects on the child's daily routine. Use open questions.

Pediatrics and geriatrics

Table 19. Average age for the acquisition of key milestones

	Motor skills	Vision and fine movement	Hearing and language	Social behavior
Newborn	Symmetrical movements, limbs flexed, head lag on pulling up	Looks at light/ faces in direct line of vision	Startles to noises/ voices	Responds to parents
Supine infant (1.5–2 months)	Raises head in prone position	Tracks objects	Cries, coos, grunts	Smiles at faces
Sitting infant (6–9 months)	6/12: sits unsupported 8/12: crawls 9/12: stands supported	6/12: 'palmar grasp' 6–7/12: transfers objects	Babbles	Develops stranger and separation anxiety. Likes playing 'peek-a-boo'
Toddler (18–24 months)	12/12: stands unsupported and makes first steps 15/12: walks 24/12: climbs stairs	12/12: 'pincer grip' 16/12: uses spoon or fork	12/12: vocabulary of 1–3 words 24/12: vocabulary of >200 words; makes phrases	Is prone to temper tantrums
Communicating child (3–4 years)	Stands on one leg. Jumps. Pedals tricycle	Mature pencil grip. Draws a circle and a cross	Makes complete sentences	Plays cooperatively with other children. Imitates parents. Achieves urinary continence

Developmental/past medical history

- Birth history:
  - maternal obstetric history
  - mode of delivery and any problems
  - gestation at delivery
  - birth weight
  - problems after birth and admission to Neonatal Intensive Care Unit
  - initial feedings
  - medical problems, childhood illnesses, immunizations
- Key milestones:
  - smiling
  - sitting
  - walking
  - talking
- Current abilities:
  - motor skills
  - vision and fine movement
  - language and hearing
  - social behavior

Systems review

Drug history

Family history

Social history

After the assessment

- Ask the parent if there is anything he/she might add that you have forgotten to ask about.
- Ask the parent if he/she has any specific questions or concerns.
- Thank the parent and child.
- Summarize your findings and offer a differential diagnosis.

Conditions most likely to come up in a developmental assessment station

- Late walker
- Developmental disorder, e.g. autism
- Mental retardation
- Emotional disorder, e.g. enuresis, elective mutism, sleep disorders
- Behavioral disorder, e.g. conduct disorder, ADHD

Neonatal examination

Specifications: A mannequin in lieu of a baby. The baby's 'mother' is also in the room.

Before starting

- Introduce yourself to the mother, explain the examination, and ask her for her consent to carry it out.
- Wash your hands.
- Ask the mother about:
  - complications of the pregnancy, if any
  - type of delivery and any complications
  - the baby's gestational age at the time of birth
  - the baby's birth weight
  - the baby's feeding, urination, and defecation
  - any concerns that she might have

The examination

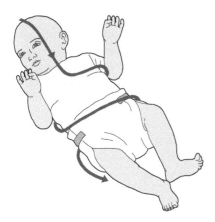

Figure 52. Neonatal examination, general order of the examination.

General inspection

Note size, color (e.g. cyanosis, jaundice), posture, tone, movements, skin abnormalities (e.g. rash, petechiae, birth marks), and any other obvious abnormalities (e.g. dysmorphic features or birth trauma such as forceps marks or chignon). Are there any signs of respiratory distress?

Head

- Palpate the anterior and posterior fontanelles for bulging (raised intracranial pressure) or depression (dehydration).
- Measure the head circumference with the tape measure passing above the ears. Head circumference in the neonate should be 33–38 cm.

Face

- Inspect the face for dysmorphological features, e.g. dysplastic or folded ears, upward slanting palpebral fissures, and a flat nasal bridge (all may be seen in Down syndrome).
- Inspect the sclerae for redness (subconjunctival hemorrhage related to birth trauma) and the irises for Brushfield spots (Down syndrome).
- Using an ophthalmoscope, test the red reflex (congenital cataracts if the red reflex is absent, retinoblastoma if instead there is a white reflex) and pupillary reflexes.
- Test eye movements (squint).
- Check the patency of the ears and nostrils.
- Elicit the rooting reflex by lightly touching a corner of the baby's mouth.
- Introduce a finger into the baby's mouth to assess the sucking reflex and the soft palate (cleft palate).
- Also examine the soft palate using a flashlight and tongue depressor.

Chest

- Inspect the chest for signs of labored breathing and for deformities, e.g. *pectus carinatum, pectus excavatum*, shield-shaped chest with widely-spaced nipples (Turner syndrome).
- Take the brachial and femoral pulses, one after the other and then both at the same time (brachio-femoral delay). Pulse rate in the neonate should be 100–160.
- Palpate the precordium and locate the apex beat.
- Auscultate the heart using the bell of your stethoscope (congenital heart defects).
- Auscultate the lungs using the diaphragm of your stethoscope. Turn the infant over and listen over the back. The respiratory rate should be less than 60 breaths per minute.

Back

- Examine the spine, focusing on the sacral pit (neural tube defects).
- Check the position and patency of the anus (anal atresia).

Abdomen

- Inspect the abdomen and the umbilical stump.
- Palpate the abdomen.
- Palpate specifically for the spleen, liver, and kidneys (thumb in front, finger in the flank), and for any masses.
- Auscultate for bowel sounds.
- Feel in the inguinoscrotal region for inguinal hernias.
- Examine the genitalia; in male infants note the position of the urethral meatus (hypospadias) and feel for the testicles (undescended testes).
- Feel for the femoral pulses.

Hips

- *Ortolani test.* With your thumbs on the inner aspects of the thighs and your index and middle fingers over the greater trochanters, flex the hips and knees to 90 degrees and then abduct the hips (an audible and palpable clunk indicates relocation of a dislocated hip).
- *Barlow test.* Next, adduct them while applying downward pressure with your thumbs (an audible and palpable clunk indicates an unstable hip that can be dislocated).

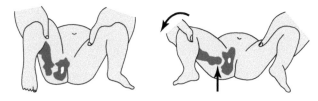

Ortolani test

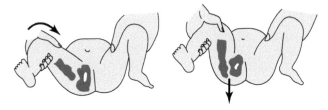

Barlow test

Figure 53. The Ortolani and Barlow tests.

Arms and hands

- Inspect the arms and hands, paying particular attention to the palmar creases (Simian crease – Down syndrome).
- Count the number of digits on each hand.

Feet

- Inspect the feet for deformities and test their range of movement.
- Count the number of digits on each foot.

Posture and reflexes

- *Head lag*. Lay the baby supine and pull up the upper body by the arms – the head should first 'lag' back, then straighten and fall forward.
- *Ventral suspension*. Hold the baby prone – the head should lie above the midline.
- *Moro or startle reflex*. Lift the head and shoulders and then suddenly drop them back – the arms and legs should abduct and extend symmetrically, and then adduct and flex (NB. some examiners may prefer that you did not test the Moro reflex).
- *Grasp reflex*. Place a finger in the baby's hand – the hand should close around your finger.

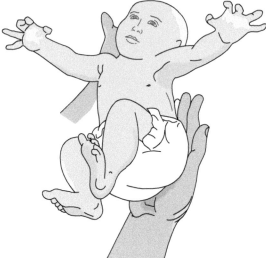

Figure 54. Eliciting the Moro reflex.

After the neonatal examination

- State that you would also measure and weigh the baby and record your findings on a growth percentile chart.
- Summarize your findings.
- Reassure the mother, if appropriate, and tell her that you are going to have the baby examined by a senior co-worker.

The six-week surveillance review

Specifications: A mannequin in lieu of a baby.

Before starting

- Introduce yourself to the parent.
- Explain the nature of the examination and obtain consent.
- Ask for the parent-held record.

The history

- Ask for the exact age, sex, and preferred name of the child.

Main concerns

- Ask if the parent has any specific concerns.

Past medical history

- Birth history:
  - pregnancy
  - gestation
  - delivery
  - birth weight
  - neonatal history
- Present health:
  - current health status
  - medication
  - social history

The examination

PART 1 – DEVELOPMENTAL ASSESSMENT

Motor skills

- Symmetrical limb movements.
- Head lag.

Vision and fine movement

- Looks at light/faces.
- Follows an object.

Hearing and language

- Responds to noises/voices.
- Normal cry.
- Ask parent if he/she is concerned about the baby's hearing.

Social behavior

- Smiles responsively.

PART 2 – PHYSICAL EXAMINATION

Growth

- Weight.
- Length.
- Head circumference.
- Plot findings on a percentile chart.

Head

- Palpate the fontanelles.

Face

- Eyes: red reflex, papillary reflexes, and eye movements (squints).
- Ears.
- Mouth – use a pen flashlight.

Chest

- Feel for the radial and femoral pulses.
- Auscultate the heart.
- Auscultate the lungs.

Back

- Examine the spine, particularly the sacral pit.

Abdomen

- Inspect and palpate the abdomen.
- Examine the external genitalia.

Hips

- Abduct the hips (Ortolani test, see *Figure 53*).
- Next, adduct them while applying downward pressure with your thumbs (Barlow test, see *Figure 53*).

After the surveillance review

- Discuss your findings with the parent.
- Use the opportunity for health promotion, e.g. immunizations, accident prevention, services available for the parents of young children.
- Elicit any remaining concerns that the parent may have.
- Thank the parent.

Pediatric examination: cardiovascular system

[Note] This station should be read in conjunction with *Station 17*.

If you are asked to examine the cardiovascular system of a younger child, be prepared to change the order of your examination and to modify your technique as appropriate. For example, you may need to examine the child on his parent's knees or auscultate his heart as soon as he stops crying. As in all pediatric stations, the quality of your rapport with the child will be of considerable importance.

Before starting

- Introduce yourself to the child and the parent.
- Explain the examination and ask for consent to carry it out.
- Position the child at 45 degrees, and ask him to remove his top(s).
- Ensure that he is comfortable.

The examination

General inspection

- From the end of the exam table, inspect the child carefully, looking for any obvious abnormalities in his general appearance and in particular for any dysmorphic features suggestive of Down syndrome (e.g. oblique eye fissures, epicanthic folds, Brushfield spots, flat nasal bridge, Simian crease), Turner syndrome (e.g. short stature, low-set ears, webbed neck, shield chest), or Marfan syndrome (e.g. tall stature, elongated limbs, *pectus carinatum* or *pectus excavatum*).
- Does the child look his age? Ask to look at the growth chart.
- Is he short of breath or cyanosed?
- Look around the child for clues such as a oxygen, PEFR meter, inhalers, etc.
- Inspect the precordium and the chest for any scars and pulsations. A median sternotomy or thoracotomy scar under the axillae may indicate the repair of a congenital heart defect such as a patent ductus arteriosus or a ventricular septal defect.

Inspection and examination of the hands

- Take both hands and assess them for:
  - color and temperature
  - clubbing
  - nail signs
- Determine the rate, rhythm, and character of both radial pulses (in younger infants, the brachial pulses). Take both femoral pulses at the same time to exclude a radiofemoral delay (coarctation of the aorta).
- Indicate that you would record the blood pressure in both arms. If you are asked to record the blood pressure, remember to use a cuff of appropriate size.

Table 20. Normal pulse rates in children	
Age in years	Pulse (beats per minute)
< 1	100–160
2–4	90–140
4–10	80–140
> 10	65–100

Inspection and examination of the head and neck

- Inspect the conjunctivae for signs of anemia or jaundice.
- Inspect the mouth and tongue for signs of central cyanosis and a high arched palate (Marfan syndrome).
- Assess the jugular venous pressure (difficult in very young infants).
- Locate the carotid pulse and assess its character.

Palpation of the heart

 Ask the child if he has any pain in the chest.

- Determine the location and character of the apex beat. In children (up to 8 years), this is found in the fourth intercostal space in the mid-clavicular line.
- Palpate the precordium for thrills and heaves.

Auscultation of the heart

 Warm up the diaphragm of your stethoscope.

- Listen for heart sounds, additional sounds, and murmurs. Using the stethoscope's diaphragm, listen in:
  - the *aortic* area
  - the *pulmonary* area
  - the *tricuspid* area
  - the *mitral* area

(See *Station 17, Figure 12.*)

- Any murmur heard must be classified according to:
  - timing
  - grading
  - site
  - radiation

Innocent murmurs are common in childhood
Innocent murmurs are:
• Systolic.
• Low-grade.
• Heard over only a relatively small area.
• Asymptomatic.

Chest examination

Auscultate the bases of the lungs and check for sacral edema.

Abdominal examination

Palpate the abdomen to exclude ascites and/or an enlarged liver. Note that the liver edge can usually be palpated in younger infants.

Peripheral pulses

Feel the temperature of the feet, palpate the femoral pulses, and check for pedal edema.

After the examination

- Cover the child.
- Ask the child and parent if they have any questions or concerns.
- Thank the child and parent.
- Indicate that you would test the urine, examine the retina with an ophthalmoscope and, if appropriate, order some key investigations, e.g. a CXR, ECG, echocardiogram.
- Summarize your findings and offer a differential diagnosis.

Conditions most likely to come up in a pediatric cardiovascular examination station
Ventricular septal defect (VSD)
• Pansystolic murmur best heard over the left lower sternal edge and possibly accompanied by a palpable thrill, parasternal heave, and displaced apex beat. Most VSDs are small and asymptomatic and may close spontaneously within the first year of life. However, a large VSD may progressively lead to higher pulmonary resistance and, finally, to irreversible pulmonary vascular changes, producing the so-called Eisenmenger syndrome (reversal of shunt to right-to-left shunt). Eisenmenger syndrome can also result from atrial septal defect and patent ductus arteriosus.
Patent ductus arteriosus (PDA)
• Continuous machine-like murmur best heard over the pulmonary area and possibly accompanied by a left subclavicular thrill, displaced apex beat, and collapsing pulse. The first heart sound is normal but the second is often obscured by the murmur. The ductus arteriosus is a shunt that runs from the pulmonary artery to the descending aorta and which enables blood to bypass the closed lungs *in utero*. A small PDA may cause no signs or symptoms and may go undetected into adulthood, but a large one can cause signs and symptoms of heart failure soon after birth.
Atrial septal defect
• Ejection systolic murmur best heard in the pulmonary area due to increased blood flow across the pulmonic valve with an associated mid-diastolic murmur best heard in the tricuspid area due to increased blood flow across the tricuspid valve. These murmurs, neither of which is particularly loud, are accompanied by a wide fixed splitting of the second heart sound and a displaced apex beat. The patient is often asymptomatic.

Pulmonary stenosis

- Loud ejection systolic murmur with an ejection click that is best heard in the pulmonary area. This murmur may be accompanied by a widely split second heart sound, and by a systolic thrill and parasternal heave. The patient is often asymptomatic.

Aortic stenosis

- Ejection systolic murmur with an ejection click best heard in the aortic area and radiating to the carotids. The murmur may be accompanied by a slow-rising pulse and a heaving cardiac apex. The patient is often asymptomatic.

Coarctation of the aorta

- Arterial hypertension in the right arm with normal to low blood pressure in the legs. There is radio-femoral delay between the right arm and the femoral artery and, in severe cases, a weak or absent femoral artery pulse. In contrast, mild cases may go undetected into adulthood.

Tetralogy of Fallot

- The tetralogy refers to VSD, pulmonary stenosis, overriding aorta, and right ventricular hypertrophy, and there may also be other anatomical abnormalities. There is cyanosis from birth or developing in the first year of life.

Pediatric examination: respiratory system

[Note] This station should be read in conjunction with *Station 22*.

If you are asked to examine the respiratory system of a younger child, be prepared to change the order of your examination and to modify your technique as appropriate. For example, you may need to examine the child on his parent's knees or auscultate his chest as soon as he stops crying. As in all pediatric stations, the quality of your rapport with the child will be of considerable importance.

Before starting

- Introduce yourself to the child and parent.
- Explain the examination and ask for consent to carry it out.
- Position the child at 45 degrees, and ask him to remove his top(s).
- Ensure that he is comfortable.

The examination

General inspection

- From the end of the exam table inspect the child carefully, looking for any obvious abnormalities in his general appearance.
- Does the child look his age? Ask to look at the growth chart.
- Is he short of breath or cyanosed?
- Is his breathing audible?
- Note the rate, depth, and regularity of his breathing.
- Look around the child for clues such as a PEFR meter, inhalers, etc.

Table 21. Normal respiratory rates in children	
Age in years	Respiratory rate (breaths per minute)
Premature infant	40–60
Term infant	30–50
6 years	19–24
12 years	16–21

Look for:

- Deformities of the chest (barrel chest, *pectus excavatum*, *pectus carinatum*) and spine.
- Asymmetry of chest expansion.
- Signs of respiratory distress such as the use of accessory muscles of respiration, suprasternal, intercostal, and/or subcostal recession, nasal flaring, and difficulty speaking.
- Added sounds such as cough, croup, wheeze, stridor.
- Harrison's sulci.
- Operative scars.

Inspection and examination of the hands

- Take both hands and assess them for color and temperature.
- Look for clubbing.

- Determine the rate, rhythm, and character of the radial pulse (in younger infants, the brachial pulse).
- State that you would record the blood pressure.

Inspection and examination of the head and neck

- Inspect the conjunctivae for signs of anemia.
- Inspect the mouth for signs of central cyanosis.
- Assess the jugular venous pressure and jugular venous pulse form.
- Palpate the cervical, supraclavicular, infraclavicular, and axillary lymph nodes.

Palpation of the chest

 Ask the child if he has any pain in the chest.

- Palpate for tracheal deviation by placing the index and middle fingers of one hand on either side of the trachea in the suprasternal notch. (As this may be uncomfortable, it is probably best omitted in younger children.)
- Palpate for the position of the cardiac apex.

[Note] Carry out all subsequent steps on the front of the chest and, once this is done, repeat them on the back of the chest.

- Palpate for equal chest expansion, comparing one side to the other.
- Palpate for tactile fremitus.

Percussion of the chest

- Percuss the chest. Start at the apex of one lung and compare one side to the other. Do not forget to percuss over the clavicles and on the sides of the chest. Note that percussion of the chest is not useful in young infants.

Auscultation of the chest

 Warm up the diaphragm of your stethoscope.

- If old enough, ask the child to take deep breaths through the mouth and, using the diaphragm of the stethoscope, auscultate the chest. Start at the apex of one lung, and compare one side to the other. Are the breath sounds vesicular or bronchial? Are there any added sounds?

Edema

- Assess for sacral and pedal edema.

After the examination

- Cover the child.
- Ask the child and parent if they have any questions or concerns.
- Thank the child and parent.
- Indicate that you would like to look at the sputum pot, measure the PEFR and, if appropriate, order some key investigations, e.g. a CXR, CBC, etc.
- Summarize your findings and offer a differential diagnosis.

Conditions most likely to come up in a pediatric respiratory examination station

Cystic fibrosis

- Autosomal recessive progressive multisystem disease that is related to a mutation in the *CFTR* gene and that leads to viscous secretions.
- In terms of the respiratory system, findings on physical examination may include delayed growth and development, finger clubbing, nasal polyps, recurrent chest infections, shortness of breath, coughing with copious phlegm production, hemoptysis, hyper-inflated chest, *cor pulmonale*.

Broncho-pulmonary dysplasia (BPD)

- Chronic lung disorder that involves inflammation and scarring in the lungs and which is most common among children who were born prematurely and who received prolonged mechanical ventilation for respiratory distress syndrome.
- Findings on physical examination may include delayed growth and development, shortness of breath, crackles, wheezes, and decreased breath sounds, hyper-inflated chest, *cor pulmonale*.

Pneumonia

- Findings on physical examination may include signs of consolidation accompanied by fever, lethargy, poor feeding, shortness of breath, productive cough, and, in some cases, hemoptysis and pleuritic chest pain.

Asthma

- Findings on physical examination may include shortness of breath, chest tightness, wheezing and coughing, signs of respiratory distress such as the use of accessory muscles of respiration and intercostal recession, hyper-inflated chest.

Pediatric examination: abdomen

[Note] This station should be read in conjunction with *Station 24*.

Before starting

- Introduce yourself to the child and parent.
- Explain the examination and ask for consent to carry it out.
- Position the child so that he is lying flat and expose his abdomen as much as possible.
- Ensure that he is comfortable.

The examination

General inspection

- From the end of the exam table, observe the child's general appearance:
  - does the child look his age? Ask to look at the growth chart
  - nutritional status
  - state of health/other obvious signs
- Inspect the abdomen noting any:
  - distension
  - localized masses
  - scars and skin changes
- Look around the child for clues such as oxygen, tubes, drains, etc.

 A distended abdomen is often a normal finding in younger infants.

Inspection and examination of the hands

- Take both hands looking for:
  - temperature and color
  - clubbing
  - nail signs
- Take the pulse.

Inspection and examination of the head, neck, and upper body

- Inspect the sclera and conjunctivae for signs of jaundice or anemia.
- Inspect the mouth, looking for ulcers (Crohn's disease), angular stomatitis (nutritional deficiency), atrophic glossitis (iron deficiency, vitamin B12 deficiency, folate deficiency), furring of the tongue (loss of appetite), and the state of the dentition.
- Examine the neck for lymphadenopathy.

Palpation of the abdomen

- Abdominal palpation can be difficult in children if they do not relax the abdominal muscles. Attempt to distract the child by handing him a toy or try to make him relax by coaxing him into palpating his abdomen and then copying his actions.

Ask the child if he has any tummy pain and keep your eyes on his face as you begin palpating his abdomen.

- *Light palpation* – begin by palpating furthest from the area of pain or discomfort and systematically palpate in the four quadrants and the umbilical area. Look for tenderness, guarding, and any masses.
- *Deep palpation* – for greater precision. Describe and localize any masses.

Palpation of the organs

- *Liver* – starting in the right lower quadrant, feel for the liver edge using the flat of your hand. Note that in younger infants the liver edge is normally palpable.
- *Spleen* – palpate for the spleen as for the liver, starting in the right lower quadrant.
- *Kidneys* – position the child close to the edge of the bed and ballot each kidney using the technique of deep bimanual palpation. Beyond the neonatal period, it is unlikely that you should be able to feel a normal kidney.

Percussion

- Percuss the liver area, also remembering to detect its upper border.
- Percuss the suprapubic area for dullness (bladder distension).
- If the abdomen is distended, test for shifting dullness (ascites).

Auscultation

- Auscultate in the mid-abdomen for abdominal sounds. Listen for 30 seconds at least before concluding that they are hyperactive, hypoactive, or absent.

Examination of the groin and genitalia

- Inspect the groin for hernias and, in boys, examine the testes (this is particularly important in younger infants).
- Note that examination of the groin and genitalia may only need to be mentioned, as it is not usually carried out in the OSCE setting.

Rectal examination

- A rectal exam is not routine practice in pediatrics and should be avoided unless specifically indicated.

After the examination

- Ask to test the urine.
- Cover the child.
- Ask the child and parent if they have any questions or concerns.
- Indicate that you would test the urine and order some key investigations, e.g. ultrasound scan, CBC, LFTs, BUN, creatinine, electrolytes, and clotting screen.
- Thank the child and parent.
- Summarize your findings and offer a differential diagnosis.

Conditions most likely to come up in a pediatric abdomen station

Constipation

- The majority of children with constipation do not have a medical disorder causing the constipation. Many things can contribute to constipation such as avoidance of the toilet (for various reasons), changes in diet or poor diet, and dehydration.
- Medical disorders that can cause chronic constipation include hypothyroidism, diabetes, cystic fibrosis, and disorders of the nervous system such as cerebral palsy and mental retardation. Constipation since birth may be from Hirschsprung disease (a.k.a. congenital aganglionic megacolon).
- Other causes of chronic constipation include depression, drug side-effects, coercive toilet training, and sexual abuse.

Celiac disease

- An autoimmune disorder of the small intestine that occurs in genetically predisposed people of all ages, but often from infancy. It is caused by a reaction to gliadin, a prolamin (gluten protein) found in wheat, barley, and rye, and results in villous atrophy.
- Symptoms include abdominal pain and cramping, diarrhea, steatorrhea, failure to thrive, and fatigue. Signs include short stature, a distended abdomen, wasted buttocks, mouth ulcers, and signs of anemia.

Kidney transplant

- A kidney transplant has been required as a consequence of end-stage renal failure, which may itself have been a consequence of a birth defect, a structural malformation, a hereditary disease such as polycystic kidney disease or Alport syndrome, a glomerular disease, or a systemic disease such as diabetes or lupus.

Pediatric examination: gait and neurological function

Before starting

- Introduce yourself to the child and parent.
- Tell the child that you are going to examine him.
- Ensure that he is comfortable.

 Examination of neurological function in children is principally a matter of observation. If the child is old enough to obey commands, a more formal assessment of gait and neurological function can be carried out, as in adults.

The examination

Neurological overview

- A brief developmental assessment should be performed to enable you to gauge the child's subsequent performance. Ask the parent the child's age and if there are any concerns about the child's vision and/or hearing.

Gait and movement

- If the child is too young to walk, observe him crawling or playing. Is he using all his limbs equally?
- If possible, observe the child walking and running. Common abnormalities of gait in children include:
  - scissoring or tiptoeing gait – suggestive of cerebral palsy or of Duchenne muscular dystrophy
  - broad-based gait: suggestive of a cerebellar disorder
  - limp – limps have many causes including dislocated hip, trauma, sepsis, and arthritis
- If possible, observe the child rising from the floor. The Gower sign (the child rising from the floor by 'climbing' up his legs) is suggestive of Duchenne muscular dystrophy.

Inspection

- Inspect all four limbs, in particular looking for muscle wasting or hypertrophy. Hypertrophy of the calves is suggestive of Duchenne muscular dystrophy.

Tone

- Assess tone and range of movement in all four limbs.
- In younger children also assess truncal tone by trying to get the child to sit unsupported.
- In young infants test head lag by lying the infant supine and pulling up his upper body by the arms.

Power

- Observe the child playing, and look for appropriate anti-gravity movement. A more formal assessment can be carried out if the child is old enough to carry out instructions.

Reflexes

- Check all reflexes as in the adult. Practice is the key!

- Note that eliciting the Babinsky sign (extensor plantar reflex) is not very discriminative in children.

Co-ordination

- If the child is old enough to carry out instructions, assess co-ordination by the finger-to-nose test or just by asking the child to jump or hop. If the child cannot carry out instructions, give him toys or some bricks and assess his co-ordination by observing him at play.

Sensation

- Indicate that you would test sensation.

Cranial nerves

- Indicate that you would test the cranial nerves – where possible this is done as in the adult.

After the examination

- Thank the parent and child.
- If appropriate, indicate that you would order some key investigations, e.g. CT, MRI, nerve conduction studies, electromyography, etc.
- Summarize your findings and offer a differential diagnosis.

Conditions most likely to appear in a pediatric gait and neurological function station
Cerebral palsy
• In most cases of cerebral palsy there is a spastic, scissoring gait. The hips, knees, and ankles are flexed, producing a crouching and tiptoeing demeanor. In addition, the hips are adducted and internally rotated, such that the knees cross or hit each other in a scissor-like movement. There is a similar pattern of flexion and adduction in the upper limbs.
Duchenne muscular dystrophy
• Severe recessive X-linked form of muscular dystrophy.
• There is rapid progression of muscle degeneration leading to generalized and symmetrical weakness of the proximal muscles.
• Symptoms and signs include muscle wasting, pseudohypertrophy of the calves, waddling gait, toe walking, frequent falls, poor endurance, difficulties running, jumping, or climbing stairs, difficulties standing unaided, and positive Gower's sign, with the child 'walking' his hands up his legs to stand upright.
Myotonic dystrophy
• Autosomal dominant progressive and highly variable multisystemic disease characterized by muscle wasting, myotonia (delayed relaxation of the muscles after voluntary contraction), cataracts, heart conduction defects, endocrine defects, and cognitive abnormalities, amongst others.
• The first muscles to be affected by wasting and weakness are typically those of the face and neck (leading to a 'fish face' and 'swan neck' appearance), hands, forearms, and feet.
• The disease commonly affects adults but it has several forms and can also present as early as birth.
Ex-premature infant

Geriatric history

Before starting

- Introduce yourself to the patient.
- Explain that you are going to ask him some questions to determine the nature of his problems, and ask for his consent to do this.
- Ensure that he is comfortable; if not, make sure that he is.
- Ask if you can take a collateral history from a caretaker.

The history

- Name, age, and past occupation if this information has not already been provided.

Chief complaint

- Enquire about the patient's chief complaint, if any. Use open questions and active listening.
- Explore any symptoms, e.g. onset, duration, previous episodes, pain, associated symptoms.
- Enquire about the effects that his symptoms are having on his everyday life.
- Elicit his ideas, concerns, and expectations.

Then aim to cover:

- Physical independence, e.g. describe a typical day.
- Functional assessment: can he stand up and walk, climb the stairs, get on and off the toilet, get in and out of the bathtub, dress, cook/clean/shop, and manage his finances and administration?
- Living arrangements: housing, heating, lighting, stairs, toileting, oven and smoke alarm, slippery bathtubs, loose rugs, adaptive or home safety aids, e.g. grab bars in the bathroom, stair lift, raised toilet seat, shower stool, bedside commode.
- Caregivers and support services.
- Social interaction: family, friends, clubs, etc. If appropriate, ask *"Who will help you if you become ill? Who should make decisions for you if you become too ill to speak for yourself?"*
- Daily diet, including nausea, vomiting, and change in appetite or weight.
- Urinary and fecal incontinence.
- Mood (e.g. *"How are you keeping in your spirits?"*). Also ask about sleep and appetite.
- Memory and cognitive impairment. Collateral information from caregiver or family member may be especially helpful in detecting cognitive impairment. For example, a positive answer to the question *'Do you think [patient's name] has been more confused lately?'* has an 80% sensitivity for delirium (*Palliat. Med.* (2010), **24**: 561–565).
- Dizziness/falls (see *Station 30: History of collapse*).
- Vision (corrective aids, accidents, difficulty reading, feeding, dressing, grooming, driving, and recognizing pills or items).

Past medical history

- Current, past, and childhood illnesses. Ask about rheumatic fever and polio.
- Surgery.

Drug history

- Prescribed medication and *compliance*. Ask also about any recent changes to the medication regimen.
- Over-the-counter drugs.
- Smoking and alcohol use.
- Allergies.

Family history

- Parents, siblings, and children. Ask specifically about diabetes, Alzheimer's disease, and cancer.

After taking the history

- Ask the patient if there is anything that he might add that you have forgotten to ask about.
- Ask if he has any questions or concerns.
- Thank him.
- Indicate that you would like to examine the patient and order some investigations.
- Formulate a problem list and suggest treatment options.

Geriatric physical examination

Examining a patient in old age (>65 years old) is very similar to examining a patient at any other age. When examining a patient in old age, important features to look out for or aspects to consider are:

Vital signs

Temperature, pulse, blood pressure (lying and standing), respiratory rate, height, weight.

General inspection

Nutritional status, posture, tremor, gait, aids.

Skin

Pressure sores, senile keratoses, senile purpura, bruises, pre-malignant or malignant lesions.

Eyes, ears, nose and throat

Vision (including fundoscopy), hearing, mouth, throat.

Musculoskeletal system

Arthritis, muscle wasting, contractures, range of motion in different joints.

Cardiovascular system

Arrhythmias, added sounds, murmurs, carotid bruits, pedal edema, absent peripheral pulses, gangrene.

Respiratory system

Chest expansion, basal crackles (may be difficult to hear because of basilar rales).

Abdomen

Organomegaly, bladder distension, abdominal aortic aneurysm, frequency and quality of abdominal sounds, rectal examination.

Breast and genitourinary

Malignancy.

Neurological examination

Tone, power, sensation, reflexes, gait, co-ordination.

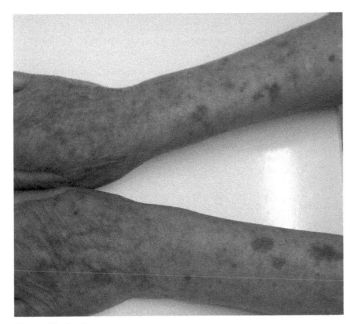

Figure 55. Senile purpura.

© Dermatlas; www.dermatlas.org – reproduced with permission.

Obstetric history

Specifications: In an exam you may be asked to focus on only a certain aspect or certain aspects of the obstetric history.

Before starting

- Introduce yourself to the patient.
- Explain that you are going to ask her some questions to uncover the nature and background of her obstetric complaint, and ask for consent to do this.
- Ensure that she is comfortable.

The history

- Name, age, and occupation.

Chief complaint

Ask about the chief complaint (if any) in some detail, e.g. onset, duration, pain, bleeding, associated symptoms, previous occurrences.

History of the present pregnancy

- Determine the duration of gestation and calculate the expected due date (EDD).
  - Ask about the date of the patient's last menstrual period (LMP).
  - Ask if her periods had been regular prior to her LMP.
  - Ask if she had been on the oral contraceptive pill (OCP). If yes, determine when she stopped taking it and the number of periods she had before becoming pregnant.
  - Determine the duration of gestation and calculate the EDD. To calculate the EDD add 9 months and 7 days to the date of the LMP. Alternatively, add 1 year, subtract 3 months, and add 7 days.
- Ask about fetal movements and, if present, about any changes in their frequency.
- Take a detailed history of the pregnancy, enquiring about:

First trimester:

  - date and method of pregnancy confirmation
  - was the pregnancy planned or unplanned? If it was unplanned, is it desired?
  - symptoms of pregnancy (e.g. sickness, indigestion, headaches, dizziness…)
  - bleeding during pregnancy
  - ultrasound scan (10–12/52)
  - chorionic villus sampling (10–13/52)

Second trimester:

  - amniocentesis (16–18/52)
  - anomaly scan (18–20/52)
  - quickening (16–18/52)

Junior Resident's tips
Dating shorthand
1/7 = one day
1/52 = one week
1/12 = one month

Third trimester:

- prenatal clinic findings – you *must* ask about blood pressure and proteinuria
- vaginal bleeding
- hospital admissions

History of previous pregnancies (past reproductive history)

Ask her if she has any children.

For each previous pregnancy, ask about:

The pregnancy, including:

- the date (year) of birth
- the duration of the pregnancy and any problems
- the mode of delivery and any problems
- the outcome

The child, including:

- the child's birth weight
- problems after birth
- the child's present condition

 Do not forget to also ask about miscarriages, stillbirths, and terminations.

Gynecological history

Take a focused gynecological history, and ask about the date and result of the last cervical smear test.

Past medical history

- Current, past, and childhood illnesses. Ask specifically about hypertension, epilepsy, diabetes and DVT.
- Surgery.
- Recent visits to the doctor.

Drug history

- Prescribed medication.
- Over-the-counter drugs.
- Folic acid supplements (should be taken from 3 months prior to conception to 3 months into pregnancy).
- Rhesus antibody injections (if required).
- Smoking.
- Alcohol use.
- Recreational drug use.
- Allergies.

Family history

- Parents, siblings, and children. Has anyone in the family ever had a similar problem?
- Is there a family history of hypertension, heart disease, or diabetes?
- *Is there a history of twins or triplets in your family or in your partner's family?*

Social history

- Support from the partner and/or family.
- Employment.
- Income and financial support.
- Housing.

After taking the history

- Ask the patient if there is anything she might add that you have forgotten to ask about.
- Thank the patient.
- If asked, summarize your findings and offer a differential diagnosis.

Conditions most likely to come up in an obstetric history station
Ectopic pregnancy
• In about 1% of pregnancies the fertilized egg implants outside the uterine cavity, most often in the Fallopian tube, but also in the cervix, ovaries, and abdomen. Clinical presentation occurs at a mean of about 7 weeks after the LMP, with a range of 5–8 weeks. Symptoms principally involve lower abdominal pain which may be worse upon moving and straining, and vaginal and internal bleeding which can be life-threatening. The principal differential is from normal pregnancy and miscarriage.
Miscarriage
• In about 15–20% of all recognized pregnancies, the pregnancy ends spontaneously at a stage when the embryo or fetus is incapable of surviving (before approximately 20–22 weeks of gestation, although most miscarriages occur prior to 13 weeks of gestation). The most common symptoms, which can range from very mild to severe, are cramping and vaginal bleeding with blood clots. The principal differential is from ectopic pregnancy.
Placenta previa
• In about 0.5% of pregnancies, usually during the second or third trimester, the placenta attaches to the uterine wall close to or covering the cervix. This classically leads to painless, bright red vaginal bleeding that increases in frequency and intensity over a period of weeks.
Placental abruption
• In about 1% of pregnancies the placenta partially or completely separates from the uterus, depriving the baby of oxygen and nutrients and causing heavy bleeding in the mother. Placental abruption can begin at any time after 20 weeks of gestation, classically with variable amounts of vaginal bleeding, abdominal pain, back pain, uterine tenderness and contraction, and rapid and repetitive uterine contractions.
False labor
Normal pregnancy

Station 64

Examination of the pregnant woman

Specifications: In an exam, most likely an anatomical model in lieu of a patient.

Before examining the patient

- Introduce yourself to the patient.
- Explain the examination and ensure consent.
- Indicate that you would weigh the patient, take her blood pressure (pre-eclampsia), dipstick her urine (pre-eclampsia, gestational diabetes) and ask her to empty her bladder.
- Position the patient so that she is lying supine (she can sit up if she finds lying supine uncomfortable).
- Ask her to expose her abdomen.
- Ensure that she is comfortable.

The examination

General inspection

Carry out a general inspection from the end of the exam table.

Inspection of the abdomen

- Abdominal distension and symmetry. Is the umbilicus everted?
- Fetal movements (after 24 weeks).
- *Linea nigra* (brownish streak running vertically along the midline from the umbilicus to the pubis).
- *Striae gravidarum* (purplish stretch marks from the current pregnancy).
- *Striae albicans* (silvery stretch marks from previous pregnancies).
- Scars.

Palpation of the abdomen

- Enquire about pain before palpating the abdomen.
- Then, facing the mother, determine the:
  - size of the uterus
  - amniotic liquor volume (normal, polyhydramnios, oligohydramnios)
  - number of fetuses
  - size of the fetus(es)
  - lie
  - presenting part
- Turning to face the mother's feet, determine the:
  - engagement

Table 22. Some important obstetric definitions
Lie. The relationship of the long axis of the fetus to that of the uterus, described as longitudinal, transverse, or oblique.
Presenting part. The part of the fetus that is in relation with the pelvic inlet, e.g. cephalic/breech for a longitudinal lie or shoulder/arm for a transverse/oblique lie.
Engagement. During engagement, the presenting part descends into the pelvic inlet in readiness for labor. Engagement is usually described in fifths of head palpable above the pelvic inlet, although sometimes the presenting part may not be the head. Engagement usually occurs after 37 weeks of gestation, before which the fetus is said to be 'floating' or 'ballotable'.

Although not usually performed, indicate that you could also determine the position, station, and attitude of the fetus. Position refers to the relationship of a point of reference on the fetus to the quadranted pelvis; station (see *Figure 56*) refers to the depth of the presenting part in relation to the ischial spines (from −5 to +5); attitude refers to the degree of flexion of the fetus' body parts.

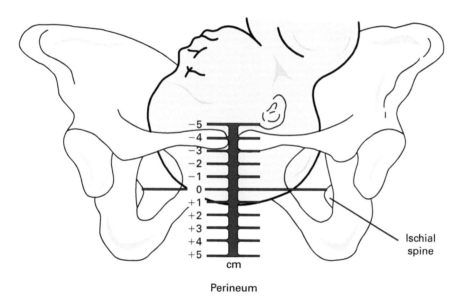

Figure 56. Measurement of station.

Symphyseal–fundal height (SFH)

Using a tape measure, measure from the mid-point of the symphysis pubis to the top of the uterus. From 20 to 38 weeks of gestation, the SFH in centimeters approximates to the number of weeks of gestation ± 2 (see *Figure 57*).

Auscultation

Classically, you can listen to the fetal heart by placing a Pinard stethoscope over the fetus' anterior shoulder and estimate the heart rate (usually 110–160 bpm). Ensure that your hands are free from the abdomen. More typically this is done using a Doppler ultrasound probe.

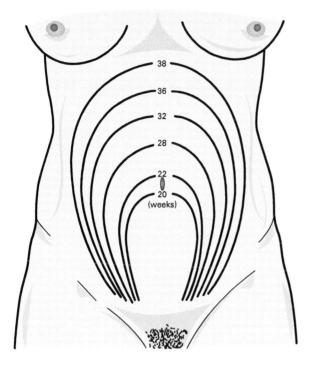

Figure 57. Expansion of the uterus during pregnancy.

After the examination

- Ask to record the blood pressure (pre-eclampsia) and to test the urine for protein (pre-eclampsia) and glucose (gestational diabetes).
- Cover the patient up.
- Thank the patient.
- Summarize your findings.

Gynecological history

Specifications: In an exam, you may be asked to circumscribe your questioning to certain aspects of the gynecological history only.

Before starting

- Introduce yourself to the patient.
- Explain that you are going to ask her some questions to uncover the nature and background of her gynecological complaint, and ask for her consent to do this.
- Ensure that she is comfortable.

The history

- Name, age, and occupation.

Chief complaint and history of presenting illness

- Ask about the chief complaint (if any) in some detail, e.g. onset, duration, pain, bleeding, associated symptoms, previous occurrences. Explore the patient's ideas, concerns and expectations. Then ask about:
  - age at menarche
  - regularity of the menses
  - dysmenorrhea
  - date of LMP – did the LMP seem normal?
  - inter-menstrual (or post-menopausal) bleeding
  - post-coital bleeding
  - vaginal discharge – if there is a vaginal discharge, ask about its amount, color, and smell. Is it causing the patient to itch?
  - date and result of the last cervical smear test
  - vaginal prolapse
  - urinary incontinence
  - coitus, present or past (*"Are you sexually active?"*)
  - dyspareunia
  - use of contraception

Past medical history

- Past gynecological history.
- Past reproductive history: previous pregnancies in chronological order, including terminations and miscarriages.
- Past medical history:
  - current, past, and childhood illnesses
  - surgery
  - recent visits to the doctor

Drug history

- – Prescribed medication, including, if appropriate, oral contraceptives and HRT.
- – Over-the-counter medication.
- – Recreational drug use.
- – Allergies.

Family history

- Ask about parents, siblings, children. Has anyone in the family had a similar problem? In the case of a suspected STD, don't forget to ask about the partner.

Social history

- Employment.
- Housing and home-help.
- Travel.
- Smoking.
- Alcohol use.

After taking the history

- Ask the patient if there is anything she might add that you have forgotten to ask about.
- Thank the patient.
- Summarize your findings and offer a differential diagnosis.

Conditions most likely to come up in a gynecological history station

Menopause

- The permanent cessation of the primary functions of the ovaries, namely, the ripening and release of ova and the release of hormones that cause both the creation and the subsequent shedding of the uterine lining. It normally occurs gradually over a period of years during the late 40s or early 50s.
- Signs and symptoms may include irregular menses, hot flushes and night sweats, increased stress, mood changes, sleep disturbances, atrophy of genitourinary tissue, vaginal dryness, and breast tenderness.

Amenorrhea

- The absence of a menstrual period in a pre-menopausal woman for a period of 3 months (or 9 months in women with a history of oligomenorrhea). It is a sign with many causes including normal pregnancy, lactation, and oral contraceptives.
- Primary amenorrhea (menstruation has not started by age 16 or age 14 if there is a lack of secondary sexual characteristics) is often related to chromosomal or developmental abnormalities.
- Secondary amenorrhea (menstruation has started but then stops) is often related to disturbances in the hypothalamo–pituitary axis due to, for example, stress, excessive dieting or exercising, PCOS, or a prolactin-secreting pituitary tumor; hypothyroidism; certain drugs such as antipsychotics and corticosteroids; intrauterine scar formation; premature menopause.

Dysmenorrhea

- Severe uterine pain possibly radiating to the back and thighs either preceding menstruation by several days or accompanying it. Associated symptoms might include menorrhagia, nausea and vomiting, diarrhea, headache, dizziness, fainting, and fatigue.
- Secondary dysmenorrhea is diagnosed in the presence of an underlying cause, commonly endometriosis or uterine fibroids.

Menorrhagia

- Abnormally heavy (>80 ml) and/or prolonged (>7 days) menstrual period at regular intervals possibly associated with dysmenorrhea and signs and symptoms of anemia. In many cases, no cause can be found. However, common causes include hormonal imbalance, pelvic inflammatory disease, endometriosis, uterine polyps or fibroids, adenomyosis, intrauterine device, coagulopathy, and certain drugs such as NSAIDs and anticoagulants.

Inter-menstrual bleeding

- Bleeding between periods may be associated with sexual intercourse or may occur spontaneously. Causes of spontaneous inter-menstrual bleeding include physiological hormone fluctuations, oral contraceptives, cervical smear test, certain drugs such as anticoagulants and corticosteroids, vaginitis, infection (e.g. chlamydia), cervicitis, cervical polyps, uterine polyps or fibroids, and adenomyosis. It is particularly important to consider cervical cancer, endometrial adenocarcinoma, threatened miscarriage, and ectopic pregnancy.

Vaginal discharge (see *Station 70*)

Dyspareunia (see *Station 70*)

Gynecological (bimanual) examination

Specifications: In an exam, a pelvic model in lieu of a patient.

Before starting

- Introduce yourself to the patient.
- Explain the examination, reassuring the patient that, although it may feel uncomfortable, it should not cause any pain.
- Obtain consent.
- Ask for a chaperone.
- Confirm that the patient has emptied her bladder.
- Indicate that you would normally carry out an abdominal examination prior to a gynecological examination.
- Ask the patient to undress, including her underwear, and to change into an examination gown. Once changed, ask the patient to lie flat on the examination table and bring her buttocks to the very edge of the table and place her feet in the stirrups. If stirrups are not available, ask her to bring her heels to her buttocks and then let her knees flop out in a 'frog-leg' position.
- Ensure that she is comfortable, and cover her up with a drape.

The examination

 Always tell the patient what you are about to do.

- Don a pair of non-sterile gloves and adjust the light source to ensure maximum visibility.
- Inspect the vulva, paying close attention to the pattern of hair distribution, the labia majora, and the clitoris. Note any redness, ulceration, masses, or prolapse.
- Palpate the labia majora for any masses.
- Try to palpate Bartholin's gland (the structure is not normally palpable).
- Lubricate the index and middle fingers of your gloved right hand.
- Use the thumb and index finger of your left hand to separate the labia minora.
- Insert the index and middle fingers of your right hand into the vagina at an angle of 45 degrees. Be sensitive to patient comfort and use only one finger to examine if the patient appears uncomfortable.
- Palpate the vaginal walls for any masses and for tenderness.
- Use your fingertips to palpate the cervix. Assess the cervix for size, shape, consistency, and mobility. Is the cervix tender? Is it open?
- Palpate the uterus: place the palmar surface of your left hand about 5 cm above the symphysis pubis and the internal fingers of your right hand behind the cervix and gently try to appose your fingers in an attempt to 'catch' the uterus. Assess the uterus for size, position, consistency, mobility, and tenderness. Can you feel any masses?

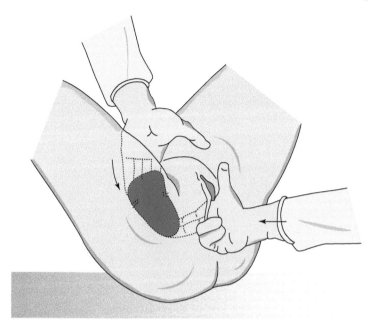

Figure 58. Technique for bimanual examination

- Palpate the right adnexae: place the palmar surface of your left hand in the right iliac fossa and the internal fingers of your right hand in the right fornix and gently try to appose your fingers in an attempt to 'catch' the ovary. Assess the ovary for any masses and for excitation tenderness (look at the patient's face).
- Use a similar technique for palpating the left adnexae.
- Once you have removed your internal fingers, inspect the glove for any blood or discharge.

After the examination

- Dispose of the gloves and wash your hands.
- Offer the patient a box of Kleenex and give her the opportunity to dress.
- Thank the patient.
- Ensure that she is comfortable.
- Indicate that you could also have carried out a speculum examination and taken a cervical smear (see *Station 67: Cervical smear test*).
- Summarize your findings and offer a differential diagnosis.

Conditions most likely to come up in gynecological examination station

Uterine fibroids

- Common and often multiple benign tumor of the smooth muscle (myometrium) of the uterus, typically found during the middle and later reproductive years. In most cases uterine fibroids are asymptomatic, but in some cases they can cause menorrhagia, dysmenorrhea, inter-menstrual bleeding, dyspareunia, urinary frequency and urgency, and fertility problems.

Ovarian cyst

- Functional fluid-filled sacs within or on the surface of an ovary. Ovarian cysts are very common, particularly in women of reproductive age, and are generally benign and asymptomatic. Symptoms can include pelvic pain, pain during urination, defecation, or sexual intercourse, urinary frequency, nausea and vomiting, abdominal fullness, breast tenderness, and menstrual irregularities.

Cervical smear test and liquid based cytology test

Specifications: An anatomical model in lieu of a patient.

Before starting

- Introduce yourself to the patient.
- Explain the procedure to her, and ask her for her consent to carry it out.
- Request a chaperone.
- Confirm that the patient has emptied her bladder.
- Ask the patient to undress, including her underwear, and to change into an examination gown. Once changed, ask the patient to lie flat on the examination table and bring her buttocks to the very edge of the table and place her feet in the stirrups. If stirrups are not available, ask her to bring her heels to her buttocks and then let her knees flop out in a 'frog-leg' position.
- Ensure that she is comfortable, and cover her up with a drape.
- Gather the appropriate equipment.

The equipment
On a tray, gather:

- non-sterile gloves
- Ayres spatula
- fixative spray (or 95% alcohol)
- bivalve speculum
- brush, if post-menopausal
- labeled slides (name, date of birth, hospital number)

The procedure

- Indicate that you would record the patient's name, date of birth, and hospital number on the slide.
- Adjust the light source to ensure maximum visibility. Many disposable speculums have a handle that can accommodate a built-in light source.
- Don the pair of gloves.
- Inspect the vulva, paying close attention to the pattern of hair distribution, the labia majora, and the clitoris. Note any redness, ulceration, masses or prolapse.
- If using a metal speculum, warm the speculum's blades in your palm.
- Place a small amount of lubricant on either side of the speculum near the tip.
- With your non-dominant hand, part the labia to ensure all hair and skin are out of the way.
- With your other hand, slowly but gently, insert the speculum with the handle facing sideways, rotating it into position (handle downward) and then opening it.
- Gently open the speculum to identify the cervix.
- Fix the speculum in the open position by tightening the screw or using the available locking mechanism.

(!) *A smear should not be taken if there is any bleeding or vaginal discharge.*

- Place the tip of the Ayres spatula in the external os and rotate the spatula by 360 degrees in either direction, all the while keeping it firmly applied to the cervix.
- Spread the material thus obtained evenly onto the labeled slides.
- Immediately spray fixative onto the slides.
- Carefully remove the speculum. Hold the speculum in the open position and completely unscrew it. Then remove the speculum slowly, rotating it sideways and allowing it to close naturally as you withdraw it.

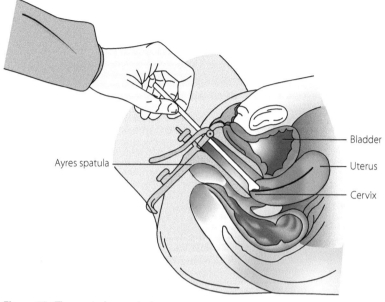

Ayres spatula

Bladder

Uterus

Cervix

Figure 59. The cervical smear test.

After the procedure

- Dispose of the speculum and the gloves.
- Offer the patient a box of Kleenex and give her the opportunity to dress.
- Meanwhile, complete an investigation form and send it off together with the labeled slide.
- Warn the patient about the possibility of spotting/bleeding after the test.
- Explain to her when and how she will receive the test results and the possible outcomes:
  - normal test – do nothing;
  - inadequate or unsatisfactory test – repeat the test;
  - abnormal test – requires human papillomavirus testing and/or colposcopy.
- Also explain when her next screening test is. Consensus guidelines suggest that pap smears should be carried out every 2 years from age 21 (or within 3 years of onset of sexual activity, whichever comes first) to 30. Between 30 and 65, women who have 3 consecutive normal smears may be screened every 3 years. Over 65, women with at least 3 normal smears and no abnormal smears in the prior 10 years may discontinue screening after discussion with their doctor.
- Ask her if she has any questions or concerns.
- Thank her.

Liquid based cytology test

Liquid based cytology (LBC) is the standard method of preparing cervical samples for examination in the laboratory, and replaces the once-conventional cervical smear test. If asked to perform an LBC test you must gather a pair of non-sterile gloves, a cervical examination brush (Cervex-Brush®), a vial containing preservative fluid, a bivalve speculum, and some water-based lubricant. Then you must carry out the following steps, the first four of which are similar to those outlined above:

- Check the expiry date on the sample collection vial and record the patient's name, date of birth and hospital number on both the vial and cytology request form.
- Adjust the light source.
- Don the pair of gloves.
- Warm, lubricate, and insert the speculum (see above).
- Insert the central bristles of the cervical brush into the endocervical canal and rotate it by 360 degrees in a clockwise direction five times.
- Immediately rinse the cervical brush in the preservative fluid by pushing it into the bottom of the vial ten times, forcing the bristles apart. Then swirl the brush vigorously to further release material.
- Inspect the cervical brush to ensure that it is free of material.
- Discard the brush.
- Carefully remove the speculum (see above).
- Tighten the cap on the vial and place it in a specimen bag, along with the request form.

Senior Resident's questions

Staging of cervical cancer

Stages are described in terms of the International Federation of Gynecology and Obstetrics (FIGO) system, which is based on clinical rather than surgical findings.

Stage 0   Carcinoma *in situ*. Tumor is present only in epithelium.

Stage I   Invasive cancer with tumor strictly confined to cervix.

Stage II   Invasive cancer with tumor extending beyond cervix or upper two-thirds of vagina, but not onto pelvic wall.

Stage III   Invasive cancer with tumor spreading to lower third of vagina or onto pelvic wall.

Stage IV   Invasive cancer with tumor spreading to other parts of the body.

NB: Various sub-stages are also described.

Breast history

Before starting

- Introduce yourself to the patient.
- Explain that you are going to ask her some questions to uncover the nature of her complaint, and ask for her consent to do this.
- Ensure that she is comfortable.

The history

- Name, age, and occupation, if this information has not already been provided. Is the patient pregnant or lactating?

Chief complaint and history of presenting illness

- Use open questions to ask about the chief complaint. Explore the patient's ideas, concerns and expectations.
- Ask specifically about pain, a lump in the breast, and nipple discharge.

For pain, determine:

- Site.
- Severity.
- Nature.
- Onset.
- Duration.
- Aggravating and alleviating factors.
- Associated signs and symptoms:
  - locally, e.g. lump, discharge, bleeding, skin changes, nipple retraction/inversion
  - systemically, e.g. tiredness, fever, night sweats, weight loss, chest or back pain
- Cyclicity.
- If the patient has had it before.
- Any other changes in the breast.

For a lump in the breast, determine:

- Site.
- Size.
- Onset.
- Duration.
- Cyclicity.
- Associated symptoms:
  - locally, e.g. pain, discharge, bleeding, skin changes, nipple retraction/inversion
  - systemically, e.g. tiredness, fever, night sweats, weight loss, chest or back pain
- If the patient has had it before.

For nipple discharge, determine:

- Amount.
- Color.
- If it is unilateral or bilateral.
- If it is from one duct or several.
- If it is spontaneous.

- Associated symptoms:
  - locally, e.g. pain, lump, bleeding, skin changes, nipple retraction/inversion
  - systemically, e.g. tiredness, fever, night sweats, weight loss, chest or back pain
- If the patient has been breast-feeding.
- If the patient has had it before.

Past medical history

- Age at menarche and (if applicable) menopause.
- Regularity of menses and date and character of LMP.
- Does the patient have any children? How old are they? Did she breast-feed them?
- Current, past, and childhood illnesses.
- Surgery.
- Previous breast investigations.
- Recent visits to the doctor.

Drug history

- Prescribed medication, especially oral contraceptives and HRT. Note that certain drugs, e.g. antipsychotics, can cause hyperprolactinemia and galactorrhea.
- Over-the-counter medications.
- Recreational drug use.
- Allergies.

Family history

- Parents, siblings, and children. Ask specifically about breast problems and cancers (especially ovarian cancer).

Social history

- Smoking.
- Alcohol use.
- Employment, past and present.
- Housing.
- Hobbies.

Systems enquiry

(If appropriate.)

After taking the history

- Ask the patient if there is anything that she might add that you have forgotten to ask about.
- Thank the patient.
- Summarize your findings and offer a differential diagnosis.
- State that you would like to examine the patient and possibly order some investigations, e.g. mammogram, ultrasound scan, fine-needle aspiration cytology (FNAC), to confirm your diagnosis.

Conditions most likely to come up in a breast history station

Fibroadenoma

- Noncancerous mass of fibrous and glandular breast tissue most commonly affecting young women and presenting as a painless, smooth, solitary, firm ('rubbery hard'), and highly mobile lump.
- Fibroadenomas can be multiple and bilateral.

Fibrocystic disease

- Common condition characterized by noncancerous lumps in the breast which can sometimes cause persistent or cyclical discomfort that peaks just before the menses. The lumps are smooth with defined edges, usually free-moving, and most often found in the upper, outer section of the breast. They may be associated with a nipple discharge that is clear, white, or green in color. The condition usually subsides after the menopause.

Mastitis

- Bacterial infection of the breast tissue, sometimes in connection with pregnancy or breast-feeding (puerperal mastitis). Signs and symptoms include fever, malaise, breast swelling and tenderness, skin redness (often in a wedge-shaped pattern), and pain or a burning sensation either persistently or only while breast-feeding. The most serious complication is breast abscess.

Breast abscess

- The lump and nearby area are red, hot, tender, and painful. Other signs and symptoms can include fever, purulent nipple discharge, and axillary lymphadenopathy. Principal complications are gangrene and septicemia.

Mammary duct ectasia

- Refers to dilatation and inflammation of a milk duct. It is most common in women in their 40s and 50s and is often asymptomatic. However, some women may have nipple discharge and breast tenderness or inflammation in the area near the nipple.

Carcinoma

- Cancer originating from breast tissue, most commonly from the inner lining of milk ducts (ductal carcinoma) or the lobules (lobular carcinoma). Signs and symptoms include an irregular breast lump or thickening, a change in the size or shape of the breast, changes to the skin over the breast such as dimpling, inverted nipple, bloody nipple discharge, and lymphadenopathy.

Intraductal papilloma

- A benign proliferation of duct epithelial cells that may present as a small painful lump in the area of the nipple. It is the most common cause of a bloody nipple discharge in young women.

Breast examination

Specifications: In an exam, you may be asked to examine a model. You may also be asked to take a brief history beforehand.

A full breast examination involves inspection, palpation of the breast tissue, palpation of the nipple, and palpation of the lymph nodes.

Before starting

- Introduce yourself to the patient.
- Explain the examination, and ask her for consent to carry it out.
- Request a chaperone.
- Ask her to undress from the waist up and hand her a gown to wear.
- Ask her to sit on the edge of the exam table, and ensure that she is comfortable.

The examination

General inspection

- From a distance, observe the patient's general appearance (age, state of health, any obvious signs).

Inspection of the breasts

- Note the size, symmetry, contour, and color of the breast; also note the pattern of venous drainage. In particular, look for the important signs of nipple inversion or retraction and *peau d'orange* (breast carcinoma). Is there a visible discharge? Are there any scars? Also remember to look under the breasts (ask the patient to lift up her breasts for you).
- Now ask the patient to put her hands atop her head and then to press them against her hips. Look for tethering and asymmetrical changes in the breast contour.

Palpation of the breasts

- Ask the patient to lie flat, because effective clinical breast examination requires flattening the breast tissue against the chest wall.
- Warm up your hands.
- Before palpating the breasts, ask if there is any breast or chest pain.
- Ask the patient to place her ipsilateral hand underneath her head.
- Starting with the normal breast, palpate the breast tissue with the palmar surface of the middle three fingers, using an even rotary movement to compress the breast tissue gently towards the chest wall. If the breasts are large, you can more effectively examine the lateral breast tissue by asking the patient to roll onto her contralateral hip while keeping her shoulders flat.
- Examine each breast using the vertical strip technique (*Figure 60*), which is the best validated.

Directions of palpation over breast surface

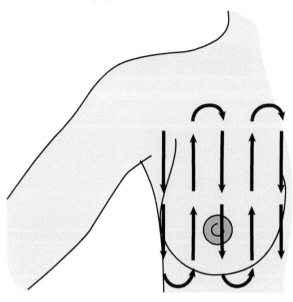

Figure 60. The vertical strip technique. Other palpation techniques include the circular and wedge techniques.

- Ask the patient to put her hands atop her head and palpate the tail of Spence between thumb and forefinger.

Assess any lump for size, shape, consistency, mobility, surface, temperature, and tenderness.

 Don't forget that there are two breasts that need examining.

Palpation of the nipple

- Hold the nipple between thumb and forefinger and gently compress it in an attempt to express a discharge (or ask the patient to do this). A discharge could signify normal lactation, galactorrhea, duct ectasia, a carcinoma, or an intraductal papilloma. Any fluid expressed should be smeared for cytology and swabbed for microbiology.

Palpation of the lymph nodes

- Expose the right axilla by lifting and abducting the arm and supporting it at the wrist with your right hand.
- With your left hand, palpate the following lymph node groups (See *Figure 51* in *Station 52*):
  - apical
  - anterior
  - posterior
  - infraclavicular and supraclavicular
  - nodes of the medial aspect of the humerus
- Now expose the left axilla by lifting and abducting the left arm and supporting at the wrist with your left hand.
- With your right hand, palpate the lymph node groups, as listed above.

Obstetrics, gynecology, and sexual health

Assess any nodes for size, shape, consistency, mobility, and tenderness.

After the examination

Indicate that you could also:

- palpate the liver edge for an enlarged liver (liver metastases)
- palpate the spine for tenderness (spinal metastases)
- auscultate the lung bases (pleural effusions)

- Cover up the patient.
- Thank the patient.
- Ensure that she is comfortable.
- Summarize your findings and offer a differential diagnosis.
- Offer further investigations if appropriate, e.g. mammogram, USS, or FNAC

Conditions most likely to come up in a breast examination station	
• Fibroadenoma	• Mammary duct ectasia
• Fibrocystic disease	• Carcinoma
• Mastitis	• Interductal papilloma
• Breast abscess	• See *Station 68* for a description of these conditions

Sexual history and HIV assessment

 This is a history that students often find difficult because of the highly personal nature of the questions involved. The trick is to remain formal and professional throughout, yet to exert tact and, if the patient becomes uncomfortable, a measure of restraint. An exam station may ask you to focus on either risk assessment or sexual function. If the latter, do not forget that sexual dysfunction often results from medical and psychiatric disorders and/or their treatments, e.g. antihypertensives, antidepressants.

The CDC recommends screening all persons who are sexually active or at high risk for HIV. High risk is defined as having sexual contact within a population in which HIV prevalence is elevated.

Before starting

- Introduce yourself to the patient.
- Set the scene: "I'd like to ask you a few questions about your sex life. Some of those are routine questions about your risk of having contracted HIV. Is that OK?"
- Reassure the patient about confidentiality.
- Explore the patient's ideas, concerns and expectations.
- Remember to be especially sensitive, tactful and empathetic.

The history and risk assessment

- Explore the patient's reason for attendance.

Sexual behavior

Structure your questions under the headings of 'Who?', 'How?', and 'Where?'

Who?

- *"Who did you last have sex with, and when was this?"*
- *"Who else have you had sex with in the last three months?"*
- *"Were they regular or casual partners?"*
- *"Do you have sex with men, women, or both?"*
- *"Do you know the HIV status of your partners?"*

How?

- *"Did you have vaginal/oral/anal sex?"*
- *"If oral or anal sex, did you give or receive it?"*
- *"Did you use protection on each occasion?"*
- If yes, *"did you have any problems with it?"*
- If no, *"when, where, how often, and with how many different partners?"*
- *"Have you ever been hurt or abused by your partner?"*

Where?

- *"Have you had sex while abroad? With whom?"*
- *"Where are your partners from?"*
- *"Is it possible that they have had sex while abroad?"*

Sexually transmitted diseases

Ask about:

- Any sores, discharge, itching, dysuria, and abdominal pain (in females). Explore any positive findings.
- History of sexually transmitted diseases (including HIV) in both the patient and his partner(s).
- In females, date and result of the last cervical smear test.

Remember that receptive anal intercourse is especially high risk for HIV.

Sexual function

- *"Do you have any problems with, or concerns about, having sex?"* You may ask specifically about erectile dysfunction and ejaculatory dysfunction in males, and about hypoactive sexual desire, anorgasmia, vaginismus, and dyspareunia in females.
- Determine the onset, course, and duration of the problem. Is the problem primary or secondary?
- Determine the frequency and timing of the problem. Is the problem partial or situational? In situational erectile dysfunction, the patient is still able to have morning erections.
- Assess the effect that the problem is having on the patient's life.

Table 23. Types of sexual dysfunction (common types are in bold)

Type of sexual dysfunction	Male	Female
Sexual desire disorders	Hypoactive sexual desire Sexual aversion (rare)	**Hypoactive sexual desire** (F > M) Sexual aversion (rare)
Sexual arousal disorders	**Erectile dysfunction***	Failure of genital response
Sexual pain disorders	Dyspareunia	Dyspareunia (F > M) Vaginismus§
Orgasm disorders	Ejaculatory impotence **Premature ejaculation****	**Anorgasmia** (F > M)

*Erectile dysfunction or impotence is more common in elderly males.

**Premature ejaculation is more common in young males engaging in their first sexual relationships.

§Vaginismus describes involuntary vaginal contractions in response to attempts at penetration.

Past medical history

- History of sexually transmitted diseases.
- History of sexual problems.
- Menstrual history: regularity of menses and date and character of LMP.
- Medical conditions. Ask specifically about hemophilia.
- Previous hospital admissions. Ask specifically if he received blood products or transfusions prior to about 1985.

Drug history

- Illicit drug use.
  - Has the patient been injecting himself?
  - If so, has he been sharing needles?
  - Do any of his partners inject themselves?

Social history

- Ask about the patient's occupation to determine if he would pose an occupational risk if HIV-positive.

After taking the history/performing the risk assessment

- Ask the patient if there is anything that he might add that you have forgotten to ask about.
- Summarize your findings and offer a further course of action, e.g. physical examination, micro-biological testing, contact tracing.
- Give him feedback on his HIV risk and, if appropriate, indicate a further course of action, e.g. an HIV test.
- Address the patient's concerns.
- Thank him.

Conditions most likely to come up in a sexual history station

Candidiasis

- Common fungal infection involving any of the *Candida* species. Infection of the vagina or vulva is often asymptomatic but may cause severe itching, burning, soreness, irritation, and a whitish or whitish-gray 'cottage cheese' discharge.
- In men, there may be red and itchy or painful sores on the penile head or foreskin. Candidiasis is not classified as an STD.

Bacterial vaginosis (BV)

- Common bacterial infection involving, amongst others, *Gardnerella vaginalis*. Although BV is not classified as an STD, it is more common in women who are sexually active and increases their susceptibility to STDs. It may be asymptomatic or there may be a thin, homogeneous, off-white, and malodorous vaginal discharge, usually in the absence of redness, itchiness, or pain.

Chlamydia

- One of the most common STDs involving the bacterium *Chlamydia trachomatis*. In women it may be asymptomatic or it might present with a yellow and odorless mucopurulent cervical discharge, dysuria, and frequency.
- In men, it is usually symptomatic, presenting with a white penile discharge with or without dysuria.
- Major complications are pelvic inflammatory disease in women, epididymitis in men, and Reiter's syndrome in both.

Gonorrhea

- A common STD caused by *Neisseria gonorrhoeae*. In women it may be asymptomatic or it might present with a greenish–yellow malodorous vaginal discharge, dysuria, and frequency.
- In men, it presents with a yellow–white penile discharge and dysuria. Symptoms typically occur 4–6 days after being infected.
- Major complications are pelvic inflammatory disease in women and epididymitis in men, or systemic spread to affect the joints and heart valves.

Trichomoniasis

- STD caused by the protozoan parasite *Trichomonas vaginalis*. Typically, only women experience symptoms but even they may be asymptomatic. Symptoms include copious amounts of a frothy, foul-smelling greenish–yellow mucopurulent discharge, itchiness, dysuria, and frequency. Discomfort may increase during intercourse and upon urination. Symptoms typically occur 5–28 days after being infected.

Syphilis

- STD caused by the bacteria *Treponema pallidum*. The disease can also be transmitted from mother to fetus, resulting in congenital syphilis. The signs and symptoms depend on which of the four stages it presents in:
  - primary stage presents at an average of 21 days after initial exposure, typically with a single chancre or
  - secondary stage presents with a diffuse rash and other symptoms
  - latent stage with few to no symptoms
  - tertiary stage with gummas, neurological, and cardiac symptoms.

Clinical Skills for Medical Students

Genital herpes

- Genital infection by herpes simplex virus (HSV) that may lead to clusters of inflamed papules and vesicles on the outer surface of the genitals or on surrounding skin. These usually appear 4–7 days after sexual exposure to HSV. Other common symptoms include pain, itching, discharge, fever, and myalgia. After 2–3 weeks, the lesions progress into ulcers and then crust and heal.

Genital warts

- Highly contagious STD caused by some sub-types of human papillomavirus (HPV), and spread through direct skin-to-skin contact during oral, genital, or anal sex. Approximately 70% of those who have sexual contact with a partner with an active infection develop genital warts, and while less than 1% of those become symptomatic, those infected can still transmit the virus.

Sexual dysfunction

- Sexual dysfunction can occur at any stage of sexual intercourse: initiation, arousal, penetration, and orgasm (see *Table 23*). It can result from organic causes (such as diabetes, angina, prostate surgery, antihypertensives, antidepressants, antipsychotics) or from psychological causes (such as depression, anxiety, sexual inexperience, traumatic sexual experience, relationship difficulties, stress), or from a combination of either.

- In secondary dysfunction there is a history of normal function, but in primary dysfunction such a history is lacking. The epidemiology of sexual dysfunction is difficult to establish, but erectile dysfunction and premature ejaculation are common in males, and anorgasmia and hypoactive sexual desire are common in females.

Condom explanation

Male and female condoms are barrier methods of contraception and prevent sperm from reaching the egg. They are very effective at preventing sexually transmitted infections but less effective than methods such as the pill in preventing pregnancy.

There are many different types of male condoms available on the market. These include plain-end or teat-end, shaped/ribbed or straight-sided, and lubricated (e.g. with inert silicone or nonoxynol-9 spermicide) condoms. Female condoms are also available, sold under the FC2 label.

Spermicidal condoms are no longer recommended as evidence suggests that nanoxynol-9 may increase the risk of HIV and other sexually transmitted infections such as chlamydia and gonorrhea.

Before starting

- Introduce yourself to the patient.
- Establish how much he already knows about using condoms. If correctly used, the male condom is 98% effective, and the female condom is 95% effective. Condoms also protect against STDs.

The equipment
• Two condoms. • A model of a penis. • An information booklet on condom use.

Explain the use of a condom

Explain that condom use should be discussed with the partner(s) and that the condom should be put on before any genital contact has taken place.

Explain/demonstrate to:

- check the expiry date
- carefully tear open the pack and remove the condom – do not use teeth or sharp nails
- position the condom on the tip of the erect penis
- squeeze out the air from the tip of the condom and gently roll it out to the base of the penis
- hold the condom at the base of the penis during penetration
- after intercourse, remove the condom ensuring that semen is not spilt
- dispose of the condom in the bin – condoms must never be re-used

Ask the patient to repeat the procedure.

 Explain that condoms can occasionally tear and that, in this event, the patient and his partner should consult a doctor or family planning clinic.

Principal side-effects are due to latex allergy and spermicide sensitivity.

Principal contraindications are oil-based lubricants such as Vaseline, hormonal vaginal creams, and antifungal preparations (Canesten is safe to use).

After the explanation

- Ask if the patient has any questions or concerns. (He may ask you about other methods of contraception.)
- Tell him to return should he have any further questions.
- Give him an information booklet on condom use.

Combined oral contraceptive pill (COCP) explanation

Before starting

- Introduce yourself to the patient.
- Ask for her name and age.
- Confirm the reason for her attendance.
- Has she considered other methods of contraception?

Explaining the COCP – items to cover

Efficacy

99.9% if used correctly, 97% in practice.

 It is important to emphasize that the pill does not protect against STDs.

Principal benefits

- More regular periods, less blood loss, fewer period pains.
- Decreased risk of ovarian cancer and endometrial cancer.
- Acne often improves.

Principal risks

- Increased risk of deep vein thrombosis and pulmonary embolism.
- Increased risk of myocardial infarction.
- Increased risk of breast cancer and adenoma of the cervix.

Principal adverse effects

- Headache.
- Nausea.
- Dizziness.
- Hypertension.
- Breast tenderness.
- Weight gain.
- Depression.

Principal contraindications

Absolute

- Thrombophlebitis, thromboembolitic disorder, or history of thromboembolism.
- Stroke.
- Ischemic heart disease.
- Liver disease.
- Kidney disease.
- History of breast cancer or other estrogen-dependent cancers of the reproductive organs.
- Pregnancy.

Relative

- Uncontrolled hypertension.
- Migraine.
- Smoking (> 15 cigarettes a day and over the age of 35).
- Abnormal vaginal bleeding.
- Sickle cell disease.
- Breast-feeding.
- Family history of hyperlipidemia, heart disease, or kidney disease.

 Remember to take a quick drug history, as many common drugs such as ampicillin or carbamazepine can alter the effectiveness of the pill.

How to take the pills

- Start taking the pill on the first Sunday after periods begin.
- Take one pill a day at the same time every day for either 21 or 28 days, depending on the number of pills in the pack.
- After finishing the 28-day pack, start another one immediately (the last seven pills in the 28-day pack are 'dummy pills').
- After finishing the 21-day pack, stop taking the pill for 7 days and then start another pack.
- Use barrier contraception during the first month on the pill.
- If you develop vomiting or diarrhea, use barrier contraception until your next period.

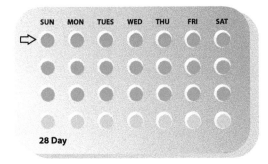

Figure 61. A 28-day pack.

What if pills are missed

If one pill is missed:

- take a pill as soon as you can remember to do so
- take the next pill at the regular time
- use barrier contraception for 7 days

If two pills are missed:

- take two pills a day for 2 days
- use barrier contraception for 7 days

If three pills are missed:

- stop taking the pill and start on another pack in 7 days' time

Before finishing

- Summarize and check understanding.
- Hand out a leaflet on the COCP.
- Tell the patient to report any severe or unexpected symptoms.

Senior Resident's questions

Other forms of contraception

Combined hormonal contraceptives are also available as a skin patch, worn for 3 out of every 4 weeks.

Low-dose progestogen-only contraceptives such as the traditional progestogen-only pill (POP, 'mini-pill'), subdermal implants (e.g. Implanon), and intrauterine systems (e.g. Mirena) inconsistently inhibit ovulation but thicken the cervical mucus and reduce sperm penetration, and also make the endometrium unsuitable for implantation. Intermediate-dose progestogen-only contraceptives such as the Cerazette pill are much more reliable at inhibiting ovulation, and high-dose progestogen-only contraceptives such as the injectable Depo-Provera inhibit ovulation completely (in the case of Depo-Provera, for up to 3 months).

The POP is taken continuously without any breaks. Whereas the COCP can be taken within a window of 12 hours, the mini-pill has a much shorter window of 3 hours. Thus, while the efficacy of the mini-pill is similar to that of the COCP, it is more dependent on user compliance. The POP is not affected by broad-spectrum antibiotics, and can often be used when the COCP is contraindicated, e.g. in smokers above the age of 35. It is contraindicated in cardiovascular disease, liver disease, breast cancer, ovarian cysts, and migraine. Side-effects, if any, are generally mild and transient. There is a small increased risk of ectopic pregnancy and breast cancer. Unlike the COCP, the POP does not regulate menstruation and can lead to either irregular menstruation or amenorrhea.

Emergency post-coital contraception comes either in the form of an intrauterine device (IUD) or an emergency contraceptive pill (ECP, 'morning-after pill') that, in contrast to medical abortion methods, act before implantation, either by postponing ovulation or by preventing implantation. The Plan B brand contains levonorgestrel which is a progestogen hormone, and is licensed for use up to 72 hours after intercourse. There is an approximate 80% reduction in the risk of pregnancy, to about 1–2% (this compares to virtually 0% for the IUD). Generally speaking, the advantages of using the ECP outweigh any theoretical or proven risks, and harm to a fetus that has already implanted is thought to be very unlikely. Side-effects include nausea, vomiting, abdominal pain, fatigue, headache, and dizziness. The ECP should not be confused with the 'abortion pill' (high dose mifepristone, RU 486).

Station 73

Pessaries and suppositories explanation

 Read in conjunction with Station 85: Explaining skills.

Like tablets, pessaries and suppositories are medication. Suppositories are for rectal use, common examples being pain-killers and steroids, whereas pessaries are for vaginal use, common examples being antibiotics and progesterone.

They are used if oral drugs cannot be given, for example, in the post-operative period or if the patient is vomiting, and if the site of action of the drug is the rectum or vagina, or near enough, for example, the colon or cervix.

In this station you may be asked to explain the use of a pessary and/or a suppository to a patient. Both scenarios have been described here.

Before starting

- Introduce yourself to the patient.
- Confirm her/his reason for attendance.
- Ask her/him if she/he has ever used a pessary or suppository before.

The explanation: items to cover

 Be sensitive to the psychological and sociocultural issues involved in placing a finger into the vagina or rectum, and be sympathetic and understanding.

Pessaries

- Pessaries are bullet-shaped medicines designed for easy insertion into the vagina using your fingers or an applicator. Your body temperature will slowly dissolve the pessary and release the medicine into your vagina.
- Wash and dry your hands.
- Remove the pessary and applicator (if supplied) from its foil or wrapper.
- If an applicator is supplied, push the pessary into the hole at its end.
- Lie down with your knees bent and legs apart.
- Carefully push the pessary high up into your vagina, pointed end first, using either your fingers or the applicator.
- If using an applicator, push the plunger to release the pessary and then remove the applicator.
- Wash your hands afterwards.
- The pessary may leak from your vagina, so it may be best to insert it before bedtime and to use a sanitary towel to avoid staining of the clothes.
- If you miss a dose, insert the pessary as soon as you remember, and then carry on as normal.
- Check the expiry date before using your pessary.
- Store in a cool, dry place and out of children's reach.
- Continue using your pessaries until the course is completed, even if this means inserting them during your monthly period.

Suppositories

- Suppositories are bullet-shaped medicines designed for easy insertion into the lower bowel (rectum) using your fingers. Your body temperature will slowly dissolve the suppository and release the medicine across your rectum and into the bloodstream.
- Empty your bowels if necessary.
- Wash and dry your hands.
- Remove the suppository from its foil or wrapper.
- Lie down on your side with one leg bent and the other straight.
- Carefully push the suppository 2–3 cm up your bottom, pointed end first, using your finger. Some people may prefer to wear a glove, but this is not necessary.
- Close your legs and lie still for a few minutes.
- Wash your hands afterwards.
- If you open your bowels within 2 hours after inserting the suppository, you need to insert another.
- The suppository may leak from your rectum, so it may be best to insert it before bedtime and (if female) to use a sanitary towel to avoid staining of the clothes.
- If you miss a dose, insert the suppository as soon as you remember, and then carry on as normal.
- Check the expiry date before using your suppository.
- Store in a cool, dark place and out of children's reach.
- Continue using your suppositories until the course is completed.

After the explanation

- Summarize and check the patient's understanding.
- Ask if she/he has any questions or concerns.
- Offer her/him a leaflet.

Rheumatological history

Before starting

- Introduce yourself to the patient.
- Explain that you are going to ask him some questions to uncover the nature of his complaint, and ask him for his consent to do this.
- Ensure that he is comfortable.

The history

Name, age, and occupation, if this information has not already been supplied.

Chief complaint

Ask the patient about the nature of his complaint. Use open questions.

Pain

Ask specifically about any pain and determine its site (i.e. which joints are affected), severity, and timing.

Stiffness

Ask specifically about stiffness and determine its site, severity and timing.

History of presenting illness

Ask about:

- The onset and any provoking factors such as trauma or infection.
- The progression.
- Any associated features:
  - local: swelling or inflammation, deformity, cracking, clicking, locking, loss of movement
  - systemic: skin problems, eye problems, GI disturbances, urethral discharge
  - general: fever, night sweats, weight loss
- Any aggravating or relieving factors such as activity, rest, NSAIDs, steroids

Social history

Ask about:

- Difficulty in completing everyday tasks and the effect that this is having on his life. If need be, you can get him to describe a typical day: getting out of bed, toileting, dressing, etc. What did he used to do that he can no longer do?
- Housing and home-help.
- Mood. Screen for the core features of depression: low mood, fatiguability, and loss of interest.
- Recent travel.

Past medical history

- Current, past, and childhood illnesses.
- Surgery.
- Recent visits to the doctor.

Drug history

- Prescribed medication, e.g. NSAIDs, steroids, immunosuppressants.
- Over-the-counter medications.
- Allergies.
- Smoking, alcohol use, and recreational drug use.

Family history

- Parents, siblings, children. Has anyone in the family ever had similar problems?

After taking the history

- Ask the patient if there is anything he might add that you have forgotten to ask about.
- Thank the patient.

Conditions most likely to come up in a rheumatological history station

Rheumatoid arthritis:

- chronic, systemic inflammatory disorder that may affect many tissues and organs, but principally the synovial joints, leading to destruction of articular cartilage and ankylosis of the joints
- women are three times more commonly affected than men
- onset is often at age 40–50, but can be at any age
- affects multiple joints, often in a symmetrical fashion, and most commonly the small joints of the hands, feet, and cervical spine
- affected joints are swollen, warm, painful, and stiff, particularly early in the morning, on waking, or following prolonged activity
- in time, there is decreased range of movement and deformity, e.g. ulnar deviation, boutonnière deformity, swan neck deformity, Z-thumb

Osteoarthritis:

- 'wear and tear' arthritis
- commonly affects the hands, feet, spine, and the large weight-bearing joints
- affected joints are painful, tender, and stiff, with symptoms worsening throughout the day and after exercise
- there may be hard bony enlargements called Heberden's nodes on the distal interphalangeal joints and Bouchard's nodes on the proximal interphalangeal joints
- there may be crepitus upon movement, restricted range of movement, joint mal-alignment, and effusions

Psoriatic arthritis:

- systemic inflammatory disorder associated with psoriasis
- asymmetrical or relatively asymmetrical arthritis most commonly affecting the distal joints in the hands and feet
- symptoms of inflammation, pain, and stiffness typically wax and wane
- there may be swelling of an entire finger or toe (dactylitis) as well as fingernail and toenail involvement

Gout:

- caused by elevated levels of urate in the blood
- more common in men
- presents as recurrent attacks of acute inflammatory arthritis
- commonly (but not exclusively) affects the metatarsal–phalangeal joint at the base of the big toe
- the joint is red, tender, hot, and swollen
- may be associated with hard, painless deposits of uric acid called tophi
- pseudogout can be difficult to distinguish from gout; it involves calcium pyrophosphate dihydrate rather than urate deposition, and it normally affects the knee and larger joints rather than the foot

Ankylosing spondylitis:

- chronic, inflammatory disorder principally affecting the axial skeleton and sacroiliac joints and potentially leading to fusion of the spine ('bamboo spine') and to damage of the spinal cord, roots, and nerves
- there is a strong genetic component
- it is more common and tends to be more severe in males
- commonly presents at ages 20–40
- morning stiffness is characteristic, and pain improves with physical activity
- may be associated with systemic features such as fever and weight loss and extra-articular manifestations such as uveitis

Septic arthritis:

- results from direct invasion of one or several joint spaces by various microorganisms, with the knee being the joint that is most commonly affected
- acute onset of joint pain with possible systemic symptoms and possible history of underlying joint disease or trauma or unprotected sexual intercourse or intravenous drug abuse
- the joint itself is red, tender, hot, and swollen, and there is often an effusion
- septic arthritis is a medical emergency

Polymyositis and dermatomyositis:

- polymyositis is an inflammatory myopathy related to dermatomyositis
- it commonly presents in early adulthood with bilateral and progressive proximal muscle weakness
- the muscles may be painful and tender and there may be systemic symptoms such as fatigue and fever
- in dermatomyositis there is also a skin rash
- the cause or causes of polymyositis and dermatomyositis is unknown

Polymyalgia rheumatica:

- muscle pain and stiffness in the neck, shoulders, and hips, especially in the morning or after inactivity
- the disorder may develop either rapidly or gradually
- systemic symptoms may include fatigue, fever, and anorexia
- there is an association with temporal arteritis
- usually affects older adults, more commonly females
- the cause of polymyalgia rheumatica is unknown
- prognosis is good, especially with corticosteroid treatment

Tendon rupture

Complications of steroid treatment

The GALS screening examination

GALS: 'Gait, arms, legs, and spine'. Remember that GALS is a screening test and that a detailed examination should therefore not be required if no positive findings are present.

Before starting

- Introduce yourself to the patient.
- Explain the examination and ask for his consent to carry it out.
- Ask him to undress to his undergarments.
- Ensure that he is comfortable.

The GALS screening examination

Brief history

- Name, age, and occupation, if this information has not already been supplied.
- *"Do you have any pain or stiffness in your muscles, back, or joints?"*
- *"Do you have any difficulty in climbing stairs?"*
- *"Do you have any difficulty washing or dressing?"*

The examination

General inspection

Inspect the patient standing. Note any obvious scars, swellings, deformities, and/or unusual posturing.

Spine

Look

- From the front.
- From behind, looking in particular for list, scoliosis and lumbar lordosis.
- From the side, looking in particular for kyphos, kyphosis and fixed flexion deformity.

Feel

- Press on each vertebral body in turn, trying to elicit tenderness.

Move

- Ask the patient to bend forward and touch his toes. Look for lumbar lordosis and for scoliosis, which should become more pronounced.

Ask him to sit down on the exam table.

- Lateral flexion of the neck. Ask him to put his ear on his shoulder and then do the same on the other side.
- Flexion and extension of the neck. Ask him to put his chin on his chest and then look up towards the ceiling.
- Spinal rotation. Ask him to turn his upper body to either side.

Demonstrate each of these movements to the patient. In particular, look for restricted range of movement and pain on movement.

Arms

Look

- Skin: rashes, nodules, nail signs
- Muscles: wasting, fasciculation
- Joints: swelling, asymmetry, deformity

 Do not forget to inspect both surfaces of the hands.

Feel

- Skin: temperature
- Muscles: general muscle bulk
- Joints: tenderness and warmth; squeeze each hand at the level of the carpal and metacarpal joints, and try to localize any tenderness by squeezing each individual joint in turn

Move

- Hands: ask the patient to squeeze your finger (grip strength); then ask him to make a pinch and attempt to 'break' his pinch (precision pinch)
- Wrists: ask him to put his hands in the prayer position and then in the reverse prayer position
- Elbows: ask him to bring up his forearms as if he were lifting weights and then to straighten out his arms alongside his body
- Shoulders: ask him to raise his arms above his head (abduction) and to then to put his hands behind his head (internal rotation); coming from below, ask him to touch his back between the shoulder blades (external rotation).

Demonstrate these movements to the patient. Look for restricted range of movement and pain on movement.

Legs

Now ask the patient to lie on the exam table.

Look

- Skin: rashes, nodules, callosities on the soles of the feet
- Muscles: wasting, fasciculation
- Joints: swelling, asymmetry, deformity

Feel

- Skin: temperature
- Joints: tenderness, warmth, and swelling; palpate each knee along the joint margin; squeeze each foot, and try to localize any tenderness by squeezing each individual joint in turn

Move

- Ask the patient to bring his heels to his bottom.
- Hold the knee and hip at 90 degrees of flexion and internally and externally rotate the hip. Keep an eye on the patient's face as you do this and ensure that you do not cause the patient unnecessary pain.
- Next, place one hand on the knee joint and extend it, feeling for any crepitus as you do so.
- Repeat on the other side.

Gait

Ask the patient to walk, observing:

- general features: rhythm, speed, stride length, limp
- the phases of gait: heel-strike, stance, push-off, and swing
- arm swing
- turning
- transfer ability: sitting and standing from a chair (note that you should already have had a chance to observe this)

After the examination

- Thank the patient.
- Offer to help the patient dress.
- Ensure that he is comfortable.
- Summarize your findings.
- If appropriate, indicate that you would perform a more detailed physical examination.

Hand and wrist examination

Before starting

- Introduce yourself to the patient.
- Explain the examination and ask for his consent to carry it out.
- Ask him to expose his arms.
- Ensure that he is comfortable.

The examination

Look

First inspect the dorsum and then the palmar surfaces of the hands.

- Skin: color, rheumatoid nodules, scars, nail changes.
- Joints: swelling, Heberden's nodes, Bouchard's nodes.
- Shape and position: normal resting position of the hand, ulnar deviation, boutonnière and swan neck deformity of the fingers, mallet finger, finger droop, Z-deformity of the thumb, muscle wasting, Dupuytren's contracture.
- Elbows: psoriatic plaques, gouty tophi, rheumatoid nodules.

Osteoarthritis: the evidence
For osteoarthritis • The presence of Heberden's or Bouchard's nodes (each has a positive LR 2)
[*Ann. Rheum. Dis.* (2009) **68:** 8–17]

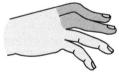 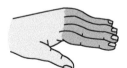

Boutonnière deformity   Swan neck deformity

Figure 62. The arthritic hand. Boutonnière and swan neck deformity of the fingers.

Feel

Ask if the hands are painful.

- Skin: temperature.
- Finger and wrist joints: swelling, synovial thickening, tenderness.
- Anatomical snuff box (fractured scaphoid).
- Tip of the radial styloid (de Quervain's disease) and head of the ulna (extensor carpi ulnaris tendinitis).

Move

Test active and passive movements, looking for limitation in the normal range of movement. Ask the patient to report any pain.

Wrist

- Flexion and extension.
- Ulnar and radial deviation.
- Pronation and supination.

Thumb

- Extension. *"Stick your thumb out to the side."*
- Abduction. *"Point your thumb up to the ceiling."*
- Adduction. *"Collect your thumb in your palm."*
- Opposition. *"Appose the tip of your thumb to the tip of your little finger."*

Fingers

Each finger should be fully extended and flexed. Look at the movements of the metacarpophalangeal and interphalangeal joints. Test the grip strength by asking the patient to make a fist and try to squeeze your fingers. Try to open the fist. Test the pincer strength by trying to break the pinch between his thumb and first finger.

Special tests

- Carpal tunnel tests:
  - try to elicit Tinel's sign by extending the hand and tapping on the median nerve in the carpal tunnel
  - try to elicit Phalen's sign by holding the hand in forced flexion for 30–60 seconds

---

Carpal tunnel syndrome: the evidence

For carpal tunnel syndrome

- Tinel's sign (positive LR 1.8, negative LR 0.8)

- Phalen's sign (positive LR 1.3, negative LR 0.7)

Although they are often taught (and thus described here), the quoted likelihood ratios make both maneuvers poor discriminatory tests for carpal tunnel syndrome.

[*JAMA* (2000) **283**: 3110–3117]

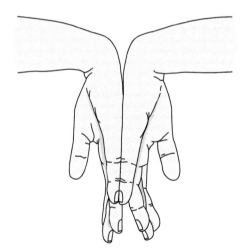

Figure 63. An alternative and quicker method for eliciting Phalen's sign.

- *Flexor profundus*: hold a finger extended at the proximal interphalangeal joint and ask the patient to flex the distal interphalangeal joint of that same finger.
- *Flexor superficialis*: ask the patient to flex a finger while holding all the other fingers on the same hand extended.
- Assess function by asking the patient to make use of an everyday object such as a pen or cup.

After the examination

- State that you would also like to examine the vascular and neurological systems of the upper limb.

- If appropriate, indicate that you would order some tests, e.g. X-ray, CBC, ESR, rheumatoid factor, etc.
- Thank the patient.
- Ensure that he is comfortable.
- Offer to help the patient put his clothes back on.
- Offer a differential diagnosis.

Conditions most likely to come up in a hand and wrist examination station

Osteoarthritis (see *Station 74*)

Rheumatoid arthritis (see *Station 74*)

Psoriatic arthritis (see *Station 74*)

Lesions of the median, radial, or ulnar nerves (see *Station 32*)

Gout (see *Station 74*)

Carpal tunnel syndrome:

- compression of the median nerve in the carpal tunnel
- more common in females
- burning pain, tingling, and numbness in the distribution of the median nerve
- possible wasting of the thenar eminence and weakness of the *abductor pollicis brevis*
- Tinel's sign and Phalen's sign are positive

Dupuytren's disease:

- fixed flexion contracture of the hand with the ring and little fingers most commonly affected
- scar tissue palpable beneath the skin of the palm with dimpling and puckering of the skin over that area

De Quervain's tenosynovitis:

- idiopathic inflammation of the tendons of *extensor pollicis brevis* and *abductor pollicis longus* muscles concerned with radial abduction of the thumb
- accompanied by difficulty gripping and pain, tenderness, and swelling over the radial styloid
- the diagnosis is verified by holding the thumb inside a clenched fist and ulnar deviating the wrist; this stretches the inflamed tendons over the radial styloid, thereby exacerbating the patient's pain (Finkelstein's test)

Trigger finger:

- idiopathic catching, snapping, or locking of the involved finger flexor tendon
- associated with pain and loss of function
- middle and ring finger most commonly affected
- the finger clicks when it is flexed and gets stuck in the flexed position
- overcoming this resistance leads to the finger snapping straight, hence the name 'trigger finger'

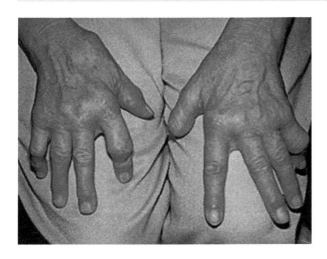

Figure 64. Rheumatoid arthritis of the hands.

Elbow examination

This station is unlikely to come up on its own but may be asked as part of a hand and wrist examination, and is included here for completeness.

Before starting

- Introduce yourself to the patient.
- Explain the examination and ask for his consent to carry it out.
- Ask him to expose his arms.
- Ensure that he is comfortable.

The examination

Look

Ask the patient to hold his arms by his side.

- Overall impression: varus or valgus deformities (look from behind), effusions, inflammation of the olecranon bursa
- Skin: rheumatoid nodules, gouty tophi, scars
- Muscle wasting: biceps, triceps, forearm

Feel

Ask if the arms are painful.

- Skin: temperature, psoriatic plaques, rheumatoid nodules, gouty tophi
- Joints: tenderness, effusions, synovial thickening. Effusions are best assessed in the triangle created by the olecranon process, radial head, and lateral epicondyle
- Bones: tenderness of the lateral and medial epicondyles

Move

- Flexion and extension:
  - tennis elbow: ask about pain at the *lateral* epicondyle on elbow *extension* and forced wrist *extension*
  - golfer's elbow: ask about pain at the *medial* epicondyle on elbow *flexion* and forced wrist *flexion*
- Pronation and supination. Show the patient how to tuck his elbows into his sides and to turn his arms so that the palm of his hands face up and down (a bit like the gesture for 'I don't know').

After the examination

- State that you would also like to examine the wrist and hand.
- State that you would also like to examine the vascular and neurological systems of the upper limb.
- If appropriate, indicate that you would order some tests, e.g. X-ray, CBC, ESR, rheumatoid factor, etc.
- Thank the patient.
- Offer to help the patient put his clothes back on.
- Ensure that he is comfortable.
- Summarize your findings and offer a differential diagnosis.

Conditions most likely to come up in an elbow examination station		
• Osteoarthritis	• Rheumatoid arthritis	• Olecranon bursitis

Shoulder examination

Before starting

- Introduce yourself to the patient.
- Explain the examination and ask for his consent to carry it out.
- Ask him to undress from the waist upward.
- Ensure that he is comfortable.

The examination

Look

Inspect from front and back.

- Overall impression: alignment, position of the arms, axillae, prominence of the acromio-clavicular and sternoclavicular joints
- Skin: color, sinuses, scars
- Muscle wasting: deltoid, periscapular muscles (supraspinatus and infraspinatus)

Feel

Ask if the shoulders are painful.

- Skin: temperature – compare both sides
- Bones and joints: palpate the bony landmarks of the shoulder, starting at the sternocla-vicular joint and moving laterally along the clavicle. Try to localize any tenderness. Can you feel any effusions?
- Biceps tendon: ask the patient to flex his arms and palpate the biceps tendon in the bicipital groove. Tenderness suggests biceps tendinitis.

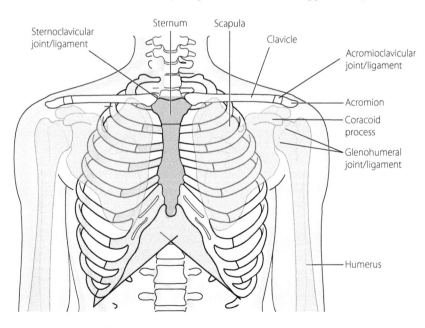

Figure 65. Anatomy of the shoulder joint.

Move

Demonstrate these movements to the patient. Note if there is a restricted range of movement and/or any pain on movement.

- Abduction: *Raise your arms above your head, making the palms of your hands touch.*
- Adduction: *Cross your arms across the front of your body.*
- Flexion: *Raise your arms forward.*
- Extension: *Pull your arms backward.*
- External rotation: *With your arms bent and your elbows tucked into your sides separate your hands.*
- Internal rotation: *With your arms bent and your elbows tucked into your sides bring your hands together.*
- Internal rotation in adduction: *Reach up your back and touch your scapulae.*
- External rotation in abduction: *Hold your hands behind your neck, like you do at the end of the day.*

 If any one movement is limited, also test the passive range of movement.

Scapular stabilizer functioning

Ask the patient to put his hands against a wall and to push against it. Observe the scapulae from behind, looking for asymmetry or winging.

After the examination

- State that you would also like to examine the vascular and neurological systems of the upper limb.
- If appropriate, indicate that you would order some tests, e.g. X-ray, CBC, ESR, rheumatoid factor, etc.
- Thank the patient.
- Offer to help the patient put his clothes back on.
- Ensure that he is comfortable.
- Summarize your findings and offer a differential diagnosis.

Conditions most likely to come up in a shoulder examination station

Frozen shoulder (adhesive capsulitis):

- the shoulder capsule becomes inflamed, resulting in pain and stiffness
- range of active movements is almost the same as that of passive movements
- the movement that is most severely restricted is external rotation
- often idiopathic
- more common in females
- rarely presents under the age of 40

Calcific tendinitis:

- pain and restricted movement result from deposits of hydroxyapatite in any tendon of the body, but most commonly in those of the rotator cuff
- pain is aggravated by elevation of the arm
- calcific deposits are visible on X-ray
- calcific tendinitis predisposes to frozen shoulder

Rotator cuff tear:

- tears of one or more of the four tendons of the rotator cuff muscles, particularly that of supraspinatus
- often asymptomatic, but may cause tenderness and pain that may radiate along the arm
- the movement that is most severely restricted is abduction; however, if the arm is passively abducted beyond 90°, the patient can abduct his arm further using the deltoid muscle

Impingement syndrome:

- impingement of the supraspinatus tendon between the acromion and the humeral head
- there is pain, weakness, and restricted movement with a painful arc of movement from 60 to 120° of abduction
- impingement syndrome predisposes to rotator cuff tear

Shoulder dislocation:

- separation of the humerus from the scapula at the glenohumeral joint
- partial separation is referred to as subluxation
- 95% of shoulder dislocations are anterior
- anterior dislocations are usually caused by the arm being forced into abduction and external rotation
- apart from a visibly displaced shoulder, there is severe pain that may radiate along the arm and a severely restricted range of movement

Bicipital tendinitis:

- inflammation of the long head of the biceps tendon, often associated with trauma or overuse
- there is shoulder pain that is exacerbated by overhead activity and by lifting
- there is tenderness over the bicipital groove
- in cases of rupture of the long head of the biceps tendon, the retracted muscle belly bulges over the anterior upper arm (Popeye sign)

Osteoarthritis (see *Station 74*)

Winging of the scapula

Referred pain from the cervical spine or the heart

Spinal examination

Before starting

- Introduce yourself to the patient.
- Explain the examination and ask for his consent to carry it out.
- Ask him to undress to his undergarments.
- Ensure that he is comfortable.

The examination

Look

Inspect from front and back.

- General inspection: ask the patient to stand and assess posture. Are there any obvious malformations?
- Skin: scars, pigmentation, abnormal hair, unusual skin creases.
- Shape and posture.
- Spine:
  - lateral curvature of the spine – *scoliosis* (observe from the back)
  - abnormal increase in the kyphotic curvature of the thoracic spine – *kyphosis* (observe from the side)
  - sharp, angular bend in the spine – a *kyphos* (observe from the side)
  - loss or exaggeration of lumbar lordosis
- Asymmetry or malformation of the chest.
- Asymmetry of the pelvis.

Feel

Ask if there is any pain.

- Palpate and percuss the spinous processes, the interspinous ligaments, and the paravertebral muscles.

Move

Ask the patient to copy your movements, looking for any limitation of range of movement. Ask the patient to indicate if any of the movements are painful.

Gait

Cervical spine

- Flexion: *Put your chin on your chest.*
- Extension: *Look at the ceiling.*
- Lateral flexion: *Put your ear onto your shoulder.*
- Rotation: *Look back over each shoulder.*

Thoracic spine

- Rotation: *Please sit down* (to stabilize the pelvis) *and twist from side to side.*

Measure chest expansion. It should be at least 5 cm.

Lumbar spine

- Flexion. *Touch your toes, keep your knees straight.*
- Extension. *Lean back, keep your knees straight.*
- Lateral flexion. *Slide your hand alongside the outside of your leg.*

Schober's test. Measure lumbar excursion by drawing a line from 10 cm above L5 to 5 cm below it and asking the patient to bend fully forward. Extension of the line by <5 cm indicates movement restriction. (Rather than drawing a line, you can just use two fingers or a measuring tape.)

Special tests

Ask the patient to lie prone.

- Palpate the sacroiliac joints for tenderness.
- Press on the mid-line of the sacrum to test if movement of the sacroiliac joints is painful.
- Femoral stretch test (L2–L4):
  - with the patient lying prone, raise the leg so as to flex the knee
  - if this does not trigger any pain, raise the leg further so as to extend the hip – pain suggests irritation of the second, third, or fourth lumbar root of that side

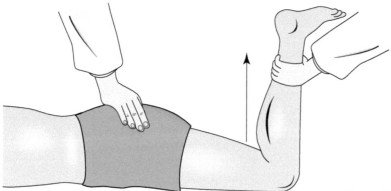

Figure 66. The femoral stretch test.

Ask the patient to lie supine.

- Straight leg raise (L5–S2):
  - with the patient lying supine, flex the hip while maintaining the knee in extension
  - pain in the thigh, buttock, and back suggests sciatica
  - the response can be amplified by concomitant dorsiflexion of the foot (Bragard's test)
  - perform Lasègue's test if you're out to impress! Flex the knee and then flex the hip to 90 degrees. With your left hand on the knee, gradually extend the knee with your right hand until the pain is reproduced. This test effectively reproduces the straight leg raise but can be performed while the patient is sitting (hip already flexed at 90 degrees requiring you to only extend the knee).

After the examination

- State that you would also like to carry out neurological and vascular examinations.
- If appropriate, indicate that you would order some tests, e.g. X-ray, MRI, DEXA, CBC, ESR, bone profile, etc.
- Thank the patient.
- Offer to help the patient put his clothes back on.
- Ensure that he is comfortable.
- Summarize your findings and offer a differential diagnosis.

Clinical Skills for Medical Students

Conditions most likely to come up in a spinal examination station

Osteoarthritis (see *Station 74*)

Ankylosing spondylitis (see *Station 74*)

Prolapsed disc:
- part of the nucleus pulposus herniates through the outer part of the disc with attending inflammation and nerve root compression
- most cases occur in the lumbar spine, most commonly at L4/L5 and L5/S1
- symptoms may include back pain that is aggravated by coughing, sneezing, or straining and relieved by lying flat; nerve root pain (often involving the sciatic nerve, 'sciatica'); other nerve root symptoms such as numbness and paresthesiae; cauda equina syndrome
- the distribution of the symptoms helps to identify the level of the lesion
- straight leg raise, Bragard's test, and Lasègue's test are positive
- commonest in men and in middle age

Muscular back pain

Scoliosis

Lumbar radiculopathy due to disc prolapse: the evidence

For lumbar radiculopathy
- A positive straight leg raise has a positive LR of 1.28 but a negative LR of 0.28. So, a negative SLR is useful in making the diagnosis of lumbar radiculopathy less likely.

[*Cochrane Database Syst. Rev.* (2010), **17**: (2)]

Hip examination

Before starting

- Introduce yourself to the patient.
- Explain the examination and ask for his consent to carry it out.
- Ask him to undress to his undergarments.
- Ensure that he is comfortable.

The examination

Look

Inspect from front and back.

- General inspection: posture, symmetry of legs and pelvis, deformity, muscle wasting, scars.
- Gait (observe from the front and back). Note any limp – antalgic, short leg, or Trendelenberg (see *Station 36*).
- Trendelenberg's test: ask the patient to stand on each leg in turn, lifting the other one off the ground by bending it at the knee. Face the patient and support him by the index fingers of his outstretched hands. The sign is positive if the pelvis drops on the non-weight bearing side.

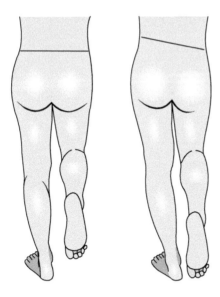

Figure 67. Negative (left) and positive Trendelenberg's test. A positive Trendelenberg's test suggests weakness of the abduction of the weight-bearing hip, and hence a problem in that hip.

Ask the patient to lie supine.

- Skin: color, sinuses, scars.
- Position: limb shortening, limb rotation, abduction or adduction deformity, flexion deformity.
- Limb length.
  - To measure *true* leg length, position the pelvis so that the iliac crests lie in the same horizontal plane, at right angles to the trunk (this is not possible if there is a fixed abduction or adduction deformity) and then measure the distance from the anterior superior iliac spine (ASIS) to the medial malleolus. True leg shortening suggests pathology of the hip joint.

- – To measure *apparent* leg length, measure the distance from the xiphisternum to the medial malleolus. Apparent leg shortening suggests pelvic tilt, most often due to an adduction deformity of the hip.
- Circumference of the quadriceps muscles at a fixed point.

Feel

Ask if there is any pain.

- Skin: temperature, effusions (difficult to feel).
- Bones and joints: bony landmarks of the hip joint, inguinal ligament.

Move

Look for limitation of the normal range of movement, and ask the patient to report any pain.

- Flexion and Thomas' test:
  - – flex both hips and place your hand in the small of the back to ensure that the lumbar lordosis has been eliminated
  - – hold one hip flexed and straighten the other leg, maintaining your hand in the small of the back – if the leg cannot be straightened and the knee is unable to rest on the exam table, a fixed flexion deformity is present
  - – repeat for the other leg
- Abduction and adduction:
  - – drop one leg over the edge of the exam table to fix the pelvis
  - – place one hand on the anterior superior iliac spine of the other leg and carry it through abduction and adduction
  - – repeat for the other leg
- Rotation:
  - – flex the hip and knee to 90 degrees
  - – hold the knee in the left hand and the ankle in the right hand
  - – using your right hand, rotate the hip internally and externally
  - – repeat for the other leg

Ask the patient to lie prone.

- Look for scars, etc.
- Feel for tenderness.
- Extend each hip in turn. Keep a hand under a bent knee and extend the hip by pulling the leg up at the ankle.

After the examination

- State that you would also like to examine the vascular and neurological systems of the lower limbs.
- If appropriate, indicate that you would order some tests, e.g. hip and knee X-ray, DEXA, CBC, ESR, bone profile, etc.
- Thank the patient.
- Offer to help the patient put his clothes back on.
- Ensure that he is comfortable.
- Summarize your findings and offer a differential diagnosis.

Conditions most likely to come up in a hip examination station

Osteoarthritis:

- the hip is held in flexion, external rotation, and adduction accompanied by pain and limited movement
- there is apparent limb shortening
- there are other signs of osteoarthritis, e.g. Heberden's nodes on the distal interphalangeal joints

Slipped capital femoral epiphysis:

- fracture through the physis resulting in slippage of the overlying epiphysis, producing a 'melting ice-cream cone' on X-ray
- limited movement of the hip, particularly internal rotation and abduction, and pain in the hip, groin, or knee
- external rotation and shortening of the affected leg
- often presents in obese prepubescent males

Trendelenburg gait (see *Station 36*)

Antalgic gait (see *Station 36*)

Hip replacement

Hip arthrodesis

Trochanteric bursitis

Clinical Skills for Medical Students

Knee examination

Before starting

- Introduce yourself to the patient.
- Explain the examination and ask for his consent to carry it out.
- Ask him to undress from the waist downward.
- Ensure that he is comfortable.

The examination

Ask the patient to stand.

Look

- Gait: observe from in front and behind, looking for instability, limp, and limited range of movement.
- Position: neutral, varus, valgus, fixed flexion.
- Squat test (avoid in elderly patients).

Ask the patient to lie supine.

- Skin: color, sinuses, scars (including arthroscopic scars).
- Shape: alignment, effusion, patellar alignment.
- Position: hyperextension, varus, valgus.

Measure quadriceps circumference a hand breadth above the patella.

Osteoarthritis of the knee: the evidence
For osteoarthritis of the knee • Bony enlargement (positive LR 10) • Restricted movement (positive LR 4)
[*Ann. Rheum. Dis.* (2010), **69**: 483–489]

Feel

Ask if there is any pain.

- Skin: temperature (compare both sides).
- Effusions: cross fluctuation, patellar tap test, and bulge test.
  - cross fluctuation: place the thumb and index finger of one hand on the joint line just below the patella and with the other hand empty the suprapatellar pouch. If an impulse is transmitted across the joint line, this indicates a large effusion.
  - patellar tap test: empty the suprapatellar pouch with one hand and dip the patella with the thumb, index finger, and middle finger of the other hand. If the patella is felt to tap the underlying bone and to bounce back up, this indicates a medium sized effusion.
  - bulge test: empty the medial parapatellar fossa by stroking the medial aspect of the joint; then empty either the suprapatellar pouch or the lateral parapatellar fossa. If the medial parapatellar fossa is seen to bulge out, this indicates a small effusion.
- Joint line at 90 degrees of flexion. Feel for any synovial thickening.
- Surrounding structures: ligaments, tibial tuberosity, femoral condyles.
- Patella: note size and height of patella and carry out patellar apprehension tests. Displace the patella laterally while flexing the knee. If the patella is unstable, the patient will either contract the quadriceps muscle or discontinue the test.

Move

- Active:
  - flexion
  - extension
- Passive:
  - flexion (to 140 degrees), feeling for crepitus and clicks
  - extension (to 0 to −10 degrees)

Special tests

- Collateral ligament tears.
  - Apply varus and valgus stresses at 0 degrees and 20 degrees of flexion. Hold the leg under one arm and apply pressure on the medial/lateral side of the knee joint.
- Cruciate ligament tears.
  - Posterior sag test: flex the knee to 90 degrees and look for a sag across the knee. The presence of a sag indicates a posterior cruciate ligament tear.
  - Anterior and posterior drawer tests: flex the knee to 90 degrees, sit on the foot (ask the patient first!), and pull the tibia back and forth. Exaggerated anterior displacement indicates that the anterior cruciate ligament is probably torn, whereas exaggerated posterior displacement indicates that the posterior cruciate ligament is probably torn.
  - Lachman's test (*Figure 68*): flex the knee to 30 degrees and, holding the thigh in one hand and the proximal tibia in the other, attempt to make the joint surfaces slide upon one another. Exaggerated anterior displacement of the tibia indicates that the anterior cruciate ligament is probably torn.

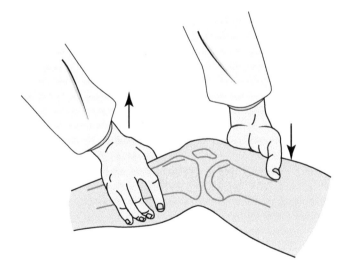

Figure 68. Lachman's test.

- Meniscal tears.
  - McMurray's test (*Figure 69*): place one hand on the knee and the other on the ankle. Flex the hip and knee. To test the medial meniscus, palpate the posteromedial margin of the joint. Then hold the leg in external rotation and extend the knee. To test the lateral meniscus, palpate the posterolateral margin of the joint. Then hold the leg in internal rotation and extend the knee. A positive test is one that elicits pain, resistance, or a reproducible click.
  - Apley's grinding test (not usually performed).

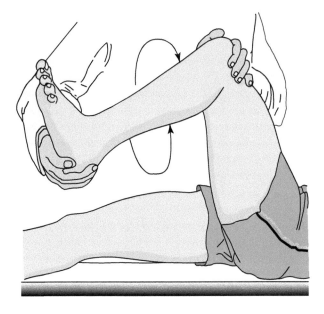

Figure 69. McMurray's test.

Lie the patient prone.

- Popliteal fossa:
  - inspect the popliteal fossa
  - palpate the popliteal fossa for a Baker's (popliteal) cyst

After the examination

- State that you would also like to examine the vascular and neurological systems of the lower limbs.
- If appropriate, indicate that you would order some tests, e.g. knee X-ray, CBC, ESR, bone profile, rheumatoid factor, etc.
- Thank the patient.
- Offer to help the patient put his clothes back on.
- Ensure that he is comfortable.
- Summarize your findings and offer a differential diagnosis.

 The age and sex of the patient have a strong bearing on the differential diagnosis.

Conditions most likely to come up in a knee examination station	
• Recurrent subluxation of the patella	• Osteoarthritis
• Chrondromalacia patellae	• Rheumatoid arthritis
• Collateral ligament tears	• Prepatellar and infrapatellar bursitis
• Cruciate ligament tears	• Baker's (popliteal) cyst
• Meniscal tears	• Tibial apophysitis (Osgood–Schlätter's disease)

Ankle and foot examination

Before starting

- Introduce yourself to the patient.
- Explain the examination and ask for his consent to carry it out.
- Ask him to undress from the waist downward.
- Ensure that he is comfortable.

The examination

The patient is standing.

Look

- General inspection: posture, symmetry, and any obvious deformities. Ask the patient to turn around.
- Gait: observe from front and back. Ask the patient to stand on his tiptoes and then on his heels.

Ask the patient to lie on the exam table.

- Skin: color, sinuses, scars, corns, calluses, ulcers.
- Shape: alignment, *pes planus* (flat foot), *pes cavus* (arched foot), deformities of the toes (*hallux valgus*, claw, hammer, and mallet toes).
- Position: varus or valgus hindfoot deformity.

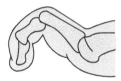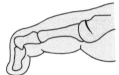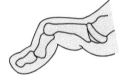

Figure 70. Claw, mallet, and hammer toes.

Feel

Ask about any pain.

- Skin: temperature (compare both sides), abnormal thickening on the soles of the feet.
- Pulses: dorsalis pedis, posterior tibial.
- Bone and joints: palpate the joint margin, forefoot (metatarsals and metatarsophalangeal joints) and hindfoot, and localize any tenderness. Remember to keep looking at the patient's face.

Move

Look for restriction of the normal range of movement. Ask the patient to report any pain.

Tibiotalar (ankle) joint

- Hold the heel in the left hand and the forefoot in the right hand.
- Plantarflex the foot (normal range 40 degrees).

- Dorsiflex the foot (normal range 25 degrees).
- Compare range of movement to that in the other foot.

Subtalar joint

- Hold the heel in the left hand and the forefoot in the right hand, as above, with the ankle fixed at 90 degrees.
- Invert the foot (normal range 30 degrees).
- Evert the foot (normal range 30 degrees).
- Compare the range of movement to that in the other foot.

Midtarsal joint

- Hold the heel in the left hand and the forefoot in the right hand.
- Flex, extend, invert, and evert the forefoot.

Toes

- Flex and extend each toe in turn. If there is any tenderness, try to localize it to a particular joint.

Ask the patient to lie prone.

- Look for any scars and for wasting of the calves.
- Palpate the calf muscle and the Achilles tendon.
- Simmond's test: squeeze the calf – if the foot plantarflexes, the Achilles tendon is intact.

After the examination

- State that you would also like to examine the vascular and neurological systems of the lower limbs.
- If appropriate, indicate that you would order some tests, e.g. foot and ankle X-ray, CBC, ESR, bone profile, rheumatoid factor, etc.
- Thank the patient.
- Offer to help the patient put his socks and shoes back on.
- Ensure that he is comfortable.
- Summarize your findings and offer a differential diagnosis.

Conditions most likely to come up in an ankle and foot examination station	
• Osteoarthritis	• Deformities of the foot
• Rheumatoid arthritis	• Plantar fasciitis
• Ankle injuries	

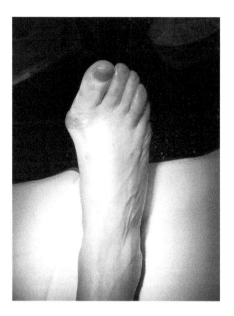

Figure 71. Hallux (abducto) valgus.

Reproduced from http://commons.wikimedia.org – photograph by Dr Henri Lelièvre.

Patient-Controlled Analgesia (PCA) explanation

In PCA, the patient presses a button to activate an infusion pump and receive a pre-prescribed intravenous bolus of analgesic, most commonly morphine or another opioid such as diamorphine, pethidine, or fentanyl.

Advantages

- Prevents delays in analgesic administration and thereby minimizes pain. In the post-operative period this may forestall a number of adverse events such as disability, pressure sores, DVT, PE, atelectasis, and constipation.
- Minimizes the amount of analgesic used, as the patient only activates the pump if he is actually in pain. Other people, such as relatives, should be told not to activate the pump.
- Provides a reliable indication of the patient's pain, and its evolution over time.
- Reduces the chance of dangerous medication errors, as the pump is programmed according to a set prescription and 'locks out' if the patient tries to activate it too often. A typical dose regimen is a 0.5–2.0 mg bolus of morphine with a lock-out of 10–15 minutes.

Disadvantages

- Patients may not receive enough analgesia (see later). In particular, patients may wake up in pain, as they cannot press the button when they are asleep. This can be circumvented by setting both a continuous rate of analgesic infusion with PRN boluses controlled by the patient.
- Patients may be physically or mentally unable to press a button.
- The pumps are expensive and may malfunction, especially if the battery is not adequately charged.

Side-effects

Side-effects of morphine include:

- respiratory depression
- sedation
- nausea and vomiting
- constipation
- urinary retention
- pruritus

Some of these side-effects can be controlled by additional prescriptions of, for example, anti-emetics, laxatives, or antihistamines. If the patient is suffering from significant respiratory depression or sedation, the dose should be decreased and alternative analgesia considered. (Remember that respiratory depression or sedation can also be caused by important post-operative complications, so do not omit to exclude these.)

Monitoring

Patients should be reviewed at regular intervals for pain, analgesic usage, and side-effects; observations should be made of the patient's pain score, analgesic usage, pulse, blood pressure, respiratory rate, and oxygen saturation. If pain relief is inadequate, the dose regime should be altered. In some cases, a continuous 'background' infusion might be considered.

Epidural analgesia explanation

Epidural analgesia, or 'epidural', is a form of regional anesthesia involving the injection of local anesthetics and/or opioids through a catheter inserted into the epidural space. Epidurals can be indicated for analgesia in labor (often simply as a matter of patient choice), for surgical anesthesia in certain operations, e.g. cesarean section, and as an adjunct to general anesthesia in others, e.g. laparatomy, hysterectomy, hip replacement. They can also be indicated for post-operative analgesia, back pain, and palliative care.

Advantages

- Permits analgesia to be delivered as a continuous infusion and/or to be patient-controlled.
- Effective and safe, with a mortality of only about 1 in 100 000.
- In post-operative analgesia, reduces the risk of certain post-operative complications such as nausea and vomiting, chest infections, and constipation.

Disadvantages

- 5% failure rate.
- In labor, increases the risk of an assisted delivery.

Contraindications

Absolute

- Raised intracranial pressure.
- Coagulopathy/anticoagulation.
- Hypovolemia.
- Skin infection at epidural site.
- Septicemia.

Relative

- Un-cooperative patient.
- Anatomical abnormalities or previous spinal surgery.
- Certain neurological disorders.
- Certain heart-valve problems.

Procedure

Epidurals are normally performed by a trained anesthetist with the patient either in the preferred sitting position or in the left lateral position. The planned entry site is identified and marked. After the skin is cleaned and local anesthetic administered, a Tuohy needle is advanced until a loss of resistance is felt anterior to the *ligamentum flavum*. The cathether, a fine plastic tube, is then threaded through the needle and the needle is removed, leaving the catheter in place. As epidurals are usually carried out in the mid-lumbar region, there is very little risk of injuring the spinal cord.

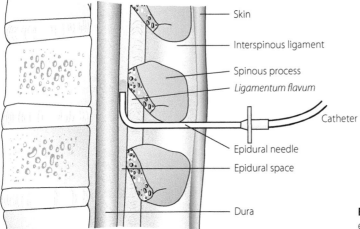

Skin

Interspinous ligament

Spinous process
Ligamentum flavum

Catheter

Epidural needle

Epidural space

Dura

Figure 72. Anatomy of the epidural space.

Side-effects and complications

- Side-effects of opioids.
- In higher doses can result in loss of other modalities of sensation (such as touch and proprioception) and motor function.
- Hypotension, most often resulting from loss of sympathetic function.
- Urinary retention.
- Accidental dural puncture resulting in a leak and a severe headache that is exacerbated by raising the head above horizontal.
- Accidental infusion into the CSF resulting in a high block or, more rarely, a total spinal involving profound hypotension, respiratory paralysis, and unconsciousness.
- Epidural hematoma that can cause spinal compression.
- Abscess formation.

Monitoring

Patients receiving epidural analgesia should be monitored for pain intensity, drug-related side-effects, and signs of complications due to the epidural procedure.

Explaining skills

These skills can be used to explain a common condition, to explain an investigation, or to explain a procedure or treatment. They can also be used in your private life, although it may then be unwise to draw a diagram or hand out a leaflet.

What to do

- Introduce yourself.
- Summarize the patient's presenting symptoms.
- Tell the patient what you are going to explain.
- Determine how much the patient already knows.
- Determine how much the patient would like to know.
- Elicit the patient's main concerns.
- Deliver the information.
  - for a medical disorder: etiology, epidemiology, clinical features, investigations/treatment, prognosis
  - for a pharmacological treatment: name, mechanism of action, procedure involved (dose, route of administration, frequency, precautions), principal benefits, principal side-effects, principal contraindications, alternatives including no treatment
  - for an investigative procedure: purpose, description of the procedure, principal risks, alternatives including no investigation, preparation required, after the procedure, results
  - for a surgical procedure: purpose, description of the procedure, principal risks, alternatives including no surgery, preparation required, anesthetic procedure, post-operative care (e.g. recovery room, oxygen, blood pressure monitoring, etc.), analgesia
- Summarize and check understanding.
- Encourage and address questions.

How to do it

- Be empathetic.
- Explore the patient's feelings.
- Give the most important information first.
- Be specific.
- Regularly check understanding.
- Pitch the explanation at the patient's level. Use simple language and short sentences. If using a medical or technical term, explain it in layman's terms.
- Use diagrams, if appropriate.
- Hand out a leaflet.
- Be honest. If you are unsure about something, say you will find out later and get back to the patient.

What not to do

- Hurry.
- Reassure too soon.
- Be patronizing.
- Give too much information.
- Use medical jargon.
- Confabulate (make things up).

"Really, now you ask me," said Alice, very much confused, "I don't think –"
"Then you shouldn't talk," said the Hatter.

Alice's Adventures in Wonderland: A Mad Tea-Party
Lewis Carroll

Some of the medical disorders, pharmacological treatments, investigative procedures, and surgical procedures that you may be asked to explain in an exam setting are listed below.

Medical disorders

- Asthma
- Diabetes
- Hypertension
- Angina
- Dementia
- Miscarriage
- Osteoarthritis/rheumatoid arthritis

Pharmacological treatments

- Statins
- Antibiotics
- Asthma inhalers
- Corticosteroids
- Insulin
- Antihypertensives
- Antidepressants
- Analgesics
- Glyceryl trinitrate
- Contraceptive pill (emergency pill, combined pill, progestogen-only preparations)
- Pessaries and suppositories
- Skin preparations, e.g. emollient, steroid cream, sunscreen

Investigative procedures

- Chest or abdominal X-ray
- CT scan
- MRI scan
- Ultrasound scan
- Echocardiography
- Flexible bronchoscopy
- Ventilation/perfusion scan
- Spirometry
- Esophagogastroduodenoscopy (EGD)

- Barium swallow/meal/follow-through
- Barium enema
- Flexible sigmoidoscopy
- Colonoscopy
- Cystoscopy

Surgical procedures

- Angioplasty
- Laparoscopic cholecystectomy
- Endoscopic retrograde cholangiopancreatography (ERCP)
- Inguinal hernia repair
- Transurethral resection of the prostate (TURP)
- Hip/knee replacement
- Varicose vein stripping

Obtaining consent

Common questions

The purpose of gaining consent

Consent is needed on every occasion a doctor wishes to initiate an investigation or treatment or any other intervention, except in emergencies or where the law dictates otherwise.

How long is consent valid for?

Consent should be seen as a continuing process rather than a one-off decision. When there has been a significant period of time between the patient agreeing to a procedure and its start, consent should be reaffirmed.

Refusal of treatment

Competent adult patients are entitled to refuse treatment even when doing so may result in permanent physical injury or death. For example, a competent Jehovah's Witness can refuse a blood transfusion even if he will surely die as a result. An adult patient is competent if he can:

- Understand what the intervention is.
- Understand why the intervention is being proposed.
- Understand the alternatives to the intervention, including no intervention.
- Understand the principal benefits and risks of the intervention and of its alternatives.
- Understand the consequences of the intervention and of its alternatives.
- Retain the information for long enough to weigh it in the balance and reach a reasoned decision, whatever that decision may be. In some cases, the patient may not have the cognitive ability or emotional maturity to reach a reasoned decision, or may be unduly affected by mental illness.

Obtaining consent

 When seeking to obtain consent, it is important not to be seen to be rattling through a list of 'must dos', but trying to elicit the patient's ideas, concerns, and expectations, and tailoring your explanations accordingly.

- The type of information that should be provided to obtain consent includes:
  - what the intervention is (use diagrams if this is helpful)
  - why the intervention is being proposed
  - alternatives to the intervention, including no intervention
  - the principal benefits and risks of the intervention and of its alternatives
  - the consequences of the intervention and of its alternatives
- Ask the patient to summarize the above information, and be certain that he is competent to give consent.
- Remind the patient that he does not have to make an immediate decision and that he can change his decision at any time.

Breaking bad news

What to do

- Introduce yourself.
- Look to comfort and privacy.
- Determine what the patient already knows.
- Determine what the patient would like to know.
- Warn the patient that bad news is coming.
- Break the bad news.
- Identify the patient's main concerns.
- Summarize and check understanding.
- Offer realistic hope.
- Arrange follow-up.
- Try to ensure there is someone with the patient when he leaves.

How to do it

- Be sensitive.
- Be empathetic.
- Maintain eye contact.
- Give information in small chunks.
- Repeat and clarify.
- Regularly check understanding.
- Give the patient time to respond. Do not be afraid of silence or of tears.
- Explore the patient's emotions.
- Use physical contact if this feels natural to you.
- Be honest. If you are unsure about something, say you will find out later and get back to the patient.

What not to do

- Hurry.
- Give all the information in one go, or give too much information.
- Use euphemisms or medical jargon.
- Lie or be economical with the truth.
- Be blunt. Words are like loaded pistols, as Jean-Paul Sartre once said.
- Prognosticate (*she's got six months, maybe seven*).

The angry patient or relative

I was angry with my friend:
I told my wrath, my wrath did end.
I was angry with my foe:
I told it not, my wrath did grow.

William Blake

The 'angry person' station can be rather unnerving, if only because medical students – and especially medical students in the earlier years of their training – are relatively sheltered from such persons.

The aim of the game is to diffuse the person's anger, *not* to ignore, placate or rationalize it. You should therefore try to be as empathetic and non-confrontational as possible.

What to do

- Introduce yourself.
- Acknowledge the person's anger.
- Try to find out the reason for his anger, e.g. frustration, fear, guilt.
- Validate his feelings.
- Let him vent his anger, or any feelings that led to his anger, e.g. frustration, fear, guilt.
- Offer to do something or for him to do something.

How to do it

- Sit at the same level as the person, not too close but not too far either.
- Make eye contact.
- Speak calmly and do not raise your voice.
- Avoid dismissive or threatening body language.
- Encourage the person to speak. Ask open rather than closed questions, and use verbal and non-verbal cues to show that you are listening.
- Empathize as much as you can.

What not to do

- Glare at the person.
- Confront him.
- Interrupt him.
- Patronize him.
- Get too close to or touch him.
- Block his exit route.
- Put the blame on others/seek to exonerate yourself.
- Make unreasonable promises.
- If the person is a patient's relative, be mindful of potential confidentiality issues.

The anxious or upset patient or relative

What to do

- Look to comfort and privacy.
- Introduce yourself and try to establish rapport.
- Acknowledge the person's emotional state, e.g. *"You seem to be very upset."*
- Explore his feelings, e.g. *"What's making you so upset?"*
- Validate his feelings, e.g. *"I think that most people would feel that way in your situation."*
- Provide honest and accurate information about the situation.
- Offer to do something or for him to do something.
- Summarize and conclude.

How to do it

- Encourage him to speak, e.g. by asking open rather than closed questions and by prompting him on, e.g. *"Can you tell me more about that?"*
- Show that you are listening, e.g. by making appropriate eye contact, adjusting your body posture, and using appropriate verbal and non-verbal cues.
- Be empathetic.
- Use silence at appropriate times. If the person sheds tears, give him the time and space to do so and hand him a Kleenex.
- Use physical contact if this feels natural to you.
- Remain poised: speak calmly, use simple sentences, and pace the information that you give.
- Repeat and clarify the information that you give, and check understanding.
- Encourage questions.

What not to do

- Ask only closed questions.
- Interrupt or rush him.
- Do all the talking.
- Dismiss or trivialize his feelings.
- Reassure too soon.
- Offer inappropriate reassurance or false hope, e.g.
  - *"There's absolutely nothing to be afraid of, everything will be just fine."*
  - *"Sure she's dead, but you'll get over her much sooner than you think."*
  - *"I'm sure your father's in a better place now."*
- If the person is a patient's relative, be mindful of potential confidentiality issues.

Station 90

Cross-cultural communication

You do not need to have a Masters in anthropology to communicate effectively with people with differing cultural or ethnic backgrounds. All you need to do is use some basic communication strategies, as detailed here. It is also important that you are seen to respect the patient's beliefs and/or values.

- Introduce yourself to the patient, and ensure that he is comfortable.
- Ask the patient's name, age, and occupation.
- Determine the patient's reason for attending.
- Elicit the patient's:
  - **I**deas
  - **C**oncerns
  - **E**xpectations
    (**ICE**)
- Establish:
  - the patient's cultural or religious group
  - the implications that this has on his reason for attending
  - the patient's individual beliefs and values
- Check that you have understood the patient's problems.
- Explore possible solutions, and agree a mutually satisfactory course of action.
- Summarize the consultation.
- Check the patient's understanding.
- Thank the patient.

Discharge planning and negotiation

Setting the scene

- Introduce yourself to the patient.
- Summarize the situation to him.
- Explore the impact that the illness/hospitalization has had on him.
- Explore his current mood and disposition.

Going home and after

- Explain that you are considering for the patient to go home.
- If a patient is going to a rehabilitation facility, specialized nursing facility, assisted living facility, or long-term acute care facility, ensure that the case management team has been involved in discharge planning.
- Elicit and address any concerns that he may have about going home. Reassure him that transport can be organized, if need be.
- Explore his home situation and support system.
- In people who are elderly or disabled, assess Activities of Daily Living (ADL): grooming, bathing, dressing, feeding, bladder, bowels, toilet use, transfer, mobility, stairs.
- Consider any extra help that can be offered to the patient, for example, social worker, home help, *meals on wheels*, health visitor, visiting nurse, specialist nurses, palliative care team, dietician, occupational therapist, speech (language) therapist, physiotherapist, psychologist, continence advisor, self-help group, day center.
- Discuss medication and compliance. Check that the patient doesn't have any concerns about taking his discharge medication and reassure him that the pharmacy can supply a pill box, if need be.
- Address risk factors. Suggest lifestyle changes that the patient may benefit from, such as stopping smoking, eating a balanced diet, exercising regularly, etc.
- Offer the patient a follow-up appointment either with his primary care physician or to help establish a new primary care provider.

Before finishing

- Summarize what has been said.
- Check the patient's understanding of what has been said.
- Ask the patient if he has any further questions or concerns.
- Thank the patient.

Appendix: Statistics

A discussion of statistical concepts doesn't typically arise when learning about history-taking and physical examination but statistics underlie much of the decision-making inherent to the diagnostic process.

The following concepts are mentioned throughout the book and understanding their application to the steps of history-taking and physical examination will help you interpret each question or probing palpation as a diagnostic test.

Sensitivity

The sensitivity of a test describes the number of people who have the disease AND have a positive test (true positive) out of all those who have the disease.

Specificity

The specificity of a test describes the number of people who do not have the disease AND have a negative test (true negative) out of all those who do not have the disease.

Likelihood ratios

The likelihood ration (LR) is a way of combining the sensitivity and specificity of a test to determine the likelihood that a positive test result or a negative test result will discriminate between those who have the disease and those who do not have the disease. Most practitioners consider a positive LR of >5 to be clinically significant.

- For a positive test, the positive likelihood ratio is the ratio of the true positive rate to false positive rate (sensitivity/1-specificity). Thus, if a test has a positive likelihood ratio of greater than 1, then a positive test is more likely to represent a true positive and a patient with a positive test is more likely to have the disease. **In practice, a positive LR of 2 or greater signifies a useful test.**
- For a negative test, the negative likelihood ratio is the ratio of the false negative rate to the true negative rate (1-sensitivity/specificity). Thus, if a test has a negative likelihood ratio of less than 1, then a negative test is more likely to represent a true negative and a patient with a negative test is more likely not to have the disease. **In practice, a negative LR of 0.5 or less signifies a useful test.**

For example, chest pain radiating to both arms simultaneously has a positive likelihood ratio of 7.1 for a myocardial infarction. Thus, a patient complaining of such symptoms is more likely to be having a myocardial infarction than not (positive LR >5).

It is important to remember that although individual exam findings or questions may have small positive or negative LRs, they should not be discounted if used in conjunction. This is because when found together, positive (or negative) results can greatly increase the likelihood of each result being a true positive. For example, the presence of PND (positive LR 2.6), a history of congestive heart failure (positive LR 5.8), and an S3 (positive LR 11) greatly increase the probability that your patient's dyspnea is caused by heart failure (positive LR of 165.88).